Circadian360

Circadian360

R. A. Massey

Hawk & Rose Publishing LLC - Michigan, U.S.A.
Book Illustrators: Robin & Ankita Mishra; Maria Hussain, Syed Omar Alee & Alex Ken; Mehran of Vector Visions
Circadian360 Logo Designer: Hamad Khan
Editor: Zobayer Shah
Typesetter/Designer: Alice Izabella

Table of Contents

Introduction

All of the information in **Circadian360** is absolutely non-secular and research-backed, derived from both a variety of sources and cultures, and this is of major importance because any individual, regardless of their faith, spirituality, background and beliefs, are able to benefit from the information in this book. This book is a universal guide for the human being seeking to reconnect with their solar blueprint, through the ongoing wisdom that has come from the practices of both our ancestors and current brothers and sisters making positive leaps forward within fields of medicine and clinical research.

The **Circadian360** book is about retuning, resetting and recalibrating the human body while honoring ourselves as light-powered vessels, and we do this by appreciating and aligning the mechanisms within us that are directly impacted by the vibrations and frequencies of the universe, our solar system, and planet. Since the onset of the 3rd Industrial Revolution, there has been a notable increase in various health issues attributed to changes in diet, food consumption, and the use of devices emitting blue light.

Research has indicated that the prevalence of obesity has risen significantly due to increased consumption of processed foods high in sugars and unhealthy fats, coupled with a decrease in physical activity levels as jobs have become more sedentary; moreover, there is growing evidence connecting the rise in depression and anxiety disorders to dietary factors, as diets high in processed foods, sugars, and low in essential nutrients have been associated with an increased risk of developing mental health issues. Cardiovascular diseases have also become more prevalent, partly due to unhealthy diets leading to conditions like high blood pressure and high cholesterol levels.

Today, the widespread use of smartphones, computers, and other devices emitting blue light have been linked to sleep disturbances and insomnia. Blue light exposure, especially during nighttime, can disrupt the production of melatonin, a hormone responsible for regulating sleep-wake cycles, and the constant use of these digital devices has also been linked to a rise in mental health issues, compounding weight upon those already living with diet and lifestyle-related anxiety and depression. This is because social media, while connecting people, has also been associated with increased feelings of social isolation, cyberbullying, and negative self-comparison, contributing to mental health challenges.

Blue light is part of the visible light spectrum of what the human eye can see, and vibrating within the 380 to 500 nanometer range, blue light has the shortest wavelength and highest energy within the visual light spectrum. In fact, the blue that humans see when we look up to the sky is…BLUE LIGHT! Yes - Sunlight is actually the biggest source of blue light, and we now know, through research, that natural blue light helps in elevating mood, boosting alertness, supporting memory and even regulating brain function.

However, according to a Cultivating Health article published in 2022 by UC Davis Health, "Constant exposure to blue light over time, especially at night, could damage retinal cells and cause vision problems such as age-related macular degeneration. It can also contribute to cataracts, eye cancer and growths on the clear covering over the white part of the eye." The article goes on to further state that, "Exposure to blue light before bedtime also can disrupt sleep patterns as it affects when our bodies create melatonin. This interruption of sleep patterns plays a role in the development of type 2 diabetes, cardiovascular disease, cancer, sleep disorders, and cognitive dysfunctions."

Confirming these statements, in an article published by Harvard Medical School's Harvard Health Publishing in 2020, 10 individuals participated in a study where their day/night sleeping patterns were modified, and startlingly, all of their blood sugar levels increased, throwing them into a prediabetic state, and their levels of leptin, a hormone that leaves people feeling full after a meal, went down; moreover, both our growing usage of and dependency on LED (Light-Emitting Diode) devices is having major ecological implications as well.

A 2022 article published by The Guardian stated that 51% of streets lights throughout the UK were already using LED lighting by the end of 2019. "The increase in blue light radiation in Europe has also reduced the visibility of stars in the night sky, which may have impacts on people's sense of nature. Blue light can also alter the behavioral patterns of animals including bats and moths, as it can change their movements towards or away from light sources." David Smith, of the conservation charity Buglife, stated: "We should consider light from a wider biological perspective [and] we must focus on better quality lighting that is harmonious with our natural world. Better quality and lower levels of lighting would help save energy, and lower financial costs, while also making our environment safer."

Personally, I wish that I could say that I've been immune to the damaging effects of artificial light and poor dietary choices, but unfortunately, like many others, it wasn't until I was EXHAUSTED from living with chronic physical and emotional weight, pain and discomforts that I decided to wake up, make changes and live my most authentic life possible!

Born in 1985, I came into the world under the blue hue of televisions and computers. My generation became the test dummies for how the internet would architect artificial worlds of addiction, reliance and compliance, through America Online Line (AOL) chatrooms, instant messaging and web browsing; simultaneously, we were also being inundated with weight-loss and dietary programs, giving rise to our horrid body image crisis in the '90's - 2000's.

When I was growing up, television was dominated by Bowflex infomercials, Suzanne Somers Thigh Master commercials, Anna-Nicole Smith endorsed TrimSpa, joyful Richard Simmons outfits, Total Gym by Chuck Norris, SlimFast ads and P90X; needless to say, as an overweight child on the borderline of a diabetes diagnosis, though the marketing tactics used by these companies weren't meant for children, the advertisements certainly made an impact on me.

Even though I had attempted to trim down my waistline by doing the 30-minute Tae Bo videotape workout in the 8th grade, by the time I weighed 260 lbs in high school, I started exploring over-the-counter fad supplements like Xenadrine, which promised weight loss. By college, I was eagerly buying bottles of Xantrex after pop music princess Britney Spears was photographed allegedly "picking up a fallen bottle from her purse."

Seeking self-improvement supplements and tools had become a hallmark of my life, because like many of you, I lived dangling off the edge of the cusp of the potential that a product, service, and/or someone else was meant to appear in my life, save me, acknowledge me in my full worth, and then somehow change my life. Knowingly and subconsciously, I was always working overtime to reach a milestone achievement, encounter and/or experience that would somehow bring about this actualized inner-self peace, purpose and existence. I was always waiting for Superman instead of living with the truth and acceptance that I am already a super being.

I would spend the next 15 years seeking knowledge, studying with herbalist mentors and gathering the works of medical professionals, gaining an appreciation for ancient self-care methods proven effective by research. Those years of growth have paved the foundation of the **Circadian360** book, and I am very proud to say that in the years since my unhealthy 20's and prior, I have been able to completely reinvent my life.

With health and wellness now being a multitrillion-dollar industry, many profit-driven programs, products, coaches and gurus don't want the world to know that our bodies are designed to thrive and not just survive! I don't want to dismiss real diseases and health conditions; however, what I am stating is that poor dietary habits, lifestyle choices, and unhealthy environments can impact our health, sometimes manifesting in various conditions. Fortunately, I have learned that some damage from these choices may be reversible through informed, healthy decisions.

A 2022 Stanford University study recruited 22 sets of identical twins, and for eight weeks, had one of each pair eat a vegan diet while the other followed a healthy omnivorous diet. *Why?* Well, even though many ancient cultures and modern advocates will attest to the fact that dietary habits have an impact upon our health, in this study, by having each set of the twins follow opposite diets while doing almost identical exercise routines (as planned by the same fitness instructor), this groundbreaking approach allowed researchers to examine how diet alone impacts health, separate from the influence of genetics and lifestyle. This was crucial to the study's success, as genetics and lifestyle are typically hard to control in human studies. Published in the JAMA Network, the study took a close look at the twins, analyzing changes in their body composition, microbiome and biological clock; moreover, all diets were approved by dietitians to be both nutritious and balanced. While many of us are fully aware of what body composition (shape, build, etc) refers to, this may be the first time that some of us are learning about both our microbiome and biological clock.

The human microbiome relates to the vast community of microorganisms, including bacteria, viruses, fungi and other microbes, living in and on the human body, and the gut microbiome specifically refers to the diverse population of microorganisms residing in the gastrointestinal tract, mainly the large intestine. Within the walls of the large intestine, this is where the gut microbiome supports and aids in digestion, producing essential vitamins, metabolizing nutrients and even helping to regulate the immune system. The biological clock (the subject at the heart of this book) relates to ancient, ancestral wisdom that has now been backed by 2017 Nobel-prize winning research. The biological clock, also known as our circadian rhythm, is an internal mechanism regulating various biological processes like sleep-wake cycles, hormone secretion, metabolism and so much more! Now, through modern science, we can actually compare our biological age relative to our chronological birth age, and knowing that health and lifestyle choices affect the aging processes in our body, this latest development in science means that we are now able to read an individual's strands of DNA and can see if their body is actually older or younger than the year that they were born.

Now, some of the results of the study are not entirely new or surprising. For example, several findings reiterate exactly what former studies on this matter have revealed: vegan diets lead to better cardiovascular health and a lower risk of heart disease than other diets.

"If you look at the (Dr. Dean) Ornish diet or the Mediterranean diet, there's definitely data showing that more plants and non-animal based sources of omega fatty acids like nuts and legumes are heart-healthy," said Dr. Diana Thiara, who leads UC San Francisco's weight management program, though she was not directly involved in the Stanford study.

At the end of the twin study, the twins on the vegan diet showed greater improvements in their health than the twins on the omnivorous diet.

The vegans had bigger declines in low-density lipoprotein cholesterol (LDL-C, often called "bad cholesterol"). In fact, the vegans' cholesterol decreased by 15.2 milligrams per deciliter (mg/dL), while the omnivores' cholesterol decreased by 2.4 mg/dL; moreover, Trimethylamine N-oxide (TMAO) plays an important role in cholesterol metabolism and metabolic stress under cholesterol overload. Higher TMAO levels are associated with an increase in unhealthy inflammation and a higher risk of heart disease. Following the 8-week study, the TMAO levels of the vegan twins were significantly lower than the omnivore twins. For one pair of female twins, the TMAO levels for the twin on the omnivore diet went up 160% and the TMAO levels for the twin on the vegan diet went down 350%!

Overall, the vegan twins on average lost 4.2 pounds more than the omnivorous twins, and the vegan twins reported a more than 20% drop in fasting insulin levels, in comparison to the omnivore twins. A high level of fasting insulin can indicate insulin resistance, a characteristic of Type 2 diabetes.

As far as the gut microbiome, Bifidobacterium, commonly found as a probiotic, is generally thought to be an anti-inflammatory exclusive to dairy that helps prevent infection and produces vitamins for the body; however, the results of the study showed that even though there was no dairy intake, the amount of Bifidobacterium actually increased more for the vegans than the omnivores. This is because we now know that having a more diverse array of plants in our dietary routines helps to both feed and are more beneficial to our microbiome than we have previously thought.

Finally, the most powerful and eye-opening data from the study were the results surrounding the impact of these diets upon the human biological clock, as researchers monitored the impact of the participant's epigenetic clocks. For clarification, while our genome or DNA is fixed, the human epigenetic clock can be changed with things like nutrition and lifestyle, and these changes then impact our biological clock and progression of our lives.

Telomeres are protective caps on the ends of stands of DNA. The length of telomeres decreases as we age. If your telomeres stay longer, you're actually in better health and have a younger biological age relative to your chronological birth age, and this means that you're actually younger than your birth year.

This is where studying these impacts on twins really showed great benefits! As twins are genetically identical, at the beginning of the study, each pair of twins had telomeres of the same length- there were no statistical differences; however, by the end of the 8-week study, in the omnivore group, there were NO changes/differences in the length of their telomeres, in comparison to the length of their telomeres at the beginning of the study. PHENOMENALLY, for the vegan twins, by the end of the study, they all had telomeres that were LONGER than their omnivore twin! <u>This means that at the end of the 8-week study, the vegan twin was biologically younger than their omnivore twin.</u>

This is such a profound and significant finding, proving that eating a vegan diet can slow or even reverse cellular aging, and this is why the content of this book is so important for all individuals; moreover, beyond shining a light on the various health and longevity benefits that can happen from both adopting a plant-based diet and realigning your biological rhythms to the sun, **Circadian360** also helps to potentially strengthen the relationship that each individual has with their own spirituality and the universe itself.

For thousands of years and longer, humans have been asking basic questions such as: *Who are we? What's the purpose and meaning of life? Is there a God?*

These existential questions are at the foundation of work being conducted by individuals, in a newer field of researched called neurotheology, where both science and the scientific method are being applied to spirituality through brain imaging studies.

Having scanned the brains of praying nuns, chanting Sikhs and meditating Buddhists, Dr. Andrew Newberg studies the relationship between the brain and religious experiences. In one study working with older individuals experiencing memory problems, Newberg took scans of their brains, then taught them a mantra-based type of meditation. He then asked them to practice that meditation for 12 minutes a day, for a total of eight weeks. At the end of the eight weeks, participants came back for another scan. As far as thinking more clearly, recalling facts and retaining memories, "They had improvements of about 10 or 15 percent," Newberg stated in an interview with National Public Radio. "This is only after eight weeks at 12 minutes a day, so you can imagine what happens in people who are deeply religious and spiritual and are doing these practices for hours a day for years and years."

I find it quite interesting that both Dr. Newberg's research into neurotheology and the previously mentioned Stanford study both showed that an individual can make a significant positive changes to their cellular health and biological age, while improving overall cognition and mental recollection, in just 8 weeks; moreover, this also reveals that making the opposing, poor dietary and lifestyle choices, for the same amount of time and/or longer, may cause an individual to live in a state of ongoing decline. Yet, the harder truth is knowing that this still doesn't change the fact that two months is also a rather long commitment to make, for many in today's modern society, especially for an individual who has never had prior experiences with embarking upon such tasks of self-improvement. It is here, at this junction of decision-making and gumption for change, where we find that the study into neurotheology is but an extension of an ongoing practice, where humans have been trying to learn more about both how the brain functions and why certain individuals behave and respond to various things differently than others.

The research in this area focuses it's attention on the frontal lobe of the brain, and we now know that the pre-frontal cortex is the part of the frontal lobe that is actually responsible for ruling over dedication, social interactions, focus, moral judgements, self-control, decisiveness, positive decision making, fairness and even how we both anticipate the future and handle ourselves in difficult situations. When the pre-frontal cortex is functioning properly, in our day to day lives, it truly acts as a "break" on impulsive and/or dangerous thoughts and behaviors.

Phineas Gage was a 19th-century railroad construction foreman who became famous in the field of neuroscience due to a traumatic accident that profoundly altered his personality and behavior.

In 1848, while working on the construction of the Rutland & Burlington Railroad in Vermont, Gage suffered a catastrophic accident. An explosion propelled à large iron rod through his skull, entering beneath his left cheekbone and exiting through the top of his head. Remarkably, Gage survived this horrific injury, but the rod had pierced through his frontal lobe, causing significant damage.

Despite the severity of the injury, Gage made an astonishing physical recovery, but his personality underwent a drastic transformation. Before the accident, Gage was described as responsible, dependable, and well-liked by his peers; however, following the injury, he became impulsive, irritable, and prone to fits of anger. He was unable to maintain employment and drifted from job to job, unable to hold down a steady position. This marked change in his behavior attracted the attention of medical professionals and scientists, leading to significant insights into the functions of the brain.

Gage's case provided crucial evidence for the localization of brain function, specifically the role of the frontal lobes in personality, decision-making, dedication and social behavior. Prior to his accident, little was known about the specific functions of different areas of the brain. Gage's case demonstrated that damage to the frontal lobe could result in profound changes in personality and behavior, effectively linking specific regions of the brain to particular cognitive functions.

In another instance, a high-ranking Salvation Army officer, married to a clergyman, experienced severe distress believing she had committed the unforgivable sin against the Holy Ghost. This conviction led to her incapacitation, rendering her unable to function normally.

After enduring years of suffering, she underwent a lobotomy, a surgical procedure that severs connections in the brain's frontal lobes. Following the operation, she became notably silent until one of her physicians inquired about her well-being and specifically asked about her beliefs regarding the Holy Ghost.

In a startling response, she smiled strangely and declared, "Oh, the Holy Ghost; there is no Holy Ghost."

Her response is both chilling and indicative of the profound impact the lobotomy had on her beliefs and perceptions. By severing communication between the frontal lobes and the rest of her brain, the lobotomy likely disrupted her cognitive and emotional processing, leading to a fundamental alteration in her understanding of religious concepts and beliefs. This case would also go on to underscore the ethical complexities surrounding lobotomy procedures and the potential for irreversible consequences on an individual's identity, beliefs, and sense of self.

Some may argue that her case proves that there is no God, 'higher power' and/or authoritative ruling energy over us; however, what is the car without its transmission in-tact and running properly? It is a car with missing and/or broken parts. This is why we must begin to see, appreciate and recognize the totality of our being and existence, giving far more grace, respect and reverence towards the vast unknowns in our lives. Remember, man-powered science is still catching up to the intuitive consciousness and spirit that is you, and we have enough research already to know that changes in brain chemistry, shape and functioning does affect an individual's perception of both themselves and the universe around them. I ask you, *"What happens to the car after an accident? What happens to the brain/body after injury?"* These accidents/changes may affect the proper functioning of either vehicle, and here's the reality: humans didn't build the human. So rather than allow this previous case to veer one's thoughts towards ruling out God, be open to understanding that the human brain's proper functioning plays a much more critical role in it's ability to thrive, connect and engage with the fabric of life itself, in ways that we still do not understand.

Finally, among the cases that shed light on the intricate relationship between personality and brain function, Pauline's story stands out vividly. Dr. Petrie, a renowned researcher who delved deeply into this connection, published an enlightening exchange with Pauline before and after her lobotomy.

Prior to the procedure, Pauline demonstrated a keen sense of moral responsibility. In a conversation prior to the procedure:

DOCTOR: What is the thing to do if you lose a watch you have borrowed from a friend?

PAULINE: Tell her. I expect you would have to pay for the loss of it.

After lobotomy, the doctor repeated the question.

DOCTOR: What is the thing to do if you lose a watch you have borrowed from a friend?

PAULINE: Borrow another watch.

From her study of many patients both before and after lobotomy, Dr. Petrie found that when, "the neural connections in the front of the brain, that is, in the frontal lobes, are severed, the individual shows a dramatic change in personality, in temperament, character, and ability. The patient after lobotomy is more satisfied with himself, with his capacities, with his style of living and style of writing, and is less preoccupied with getting things just right; his standards have dropped."

Based on Dr. Petrie's findings, it is fair to say that this may even be considered mental regression, with the individual becoming incapable of accessing higher levels of thought, being and action, almost to a point of returning to basic acts of survival. So it is not just that the frontal lobe of the human brain affects an individual's dedication to tasks, social interactions, ability to focus, moral judgements, self-control, positive decision-making, fairness and overall character, it also is the determining factors by which each person is able to assess, care for and nurture both their moral character and connection to a "higher authority"; moreover, blunt, injurious brain trauma doesn't have to be inflicted upon the frontal lobe for damage to be done, in order to cause levels of impairment.

In addition to smoking and both drug and alcohol abuse, a diet high in processed foods, sugar, and unhealthy fats can contribute to inflammation and oxidative stress in the brain, which may negatively impact frontal lobe function. Nutrient deficiencies, such as low levels of omega-3 fatty acids, vitamins, and minerals, can also impair cognitive function and brain health. Also, sedentary behavior like sitting all day and a lack of regular exercise can have detrimental effects on brain health, including reduced blood flow to the frontal lobes and decreased production of neurotrophic factors essential for neuronal growth and connectivity.

Sadly, in today's world, even those who maintain healthy eating habits and avoid the consumption of alcohol and drugs are still living with chronic stress and sleep deprivation.

Studies have revealed that prolonged exposure to stress can lead to dysregulation of the hypothalamic-pituitary-adrenal (HPA) axis in our brains and the excessive release of stress hormones like cortisol. Chronic stress eventually can damage neurons in the frontal lobes and prefrontal cortex, impairing cognitive function, decision-making, and emotional regulation; moreover, when one is constantly stressed, they aren't also maintaining a good sleep schedule. This only makes matters worse, as inadequate sleep or poor sleep quality can disrupt neural activity in the frontal lobes and prefrontal cortex, impairing executive function, attention, and memory. Chronic sleep deprivation has also been associated with cognitive deficits and an increased risk of mental health disorders.

A recent study showed that a 1/3 of adults and 1/2 of all individuals under the age of 30 are now waking up at night to check their phones; moreover, some individuals are reporting that they don't even have a memory of waking up and checking their phones after they've done it! This is alarming and scary.

Across the board, it is clear that what we eat, when we eat, how we engage with artificial light sources, when we rest/sleep and how we allocate our daylight hours are all inextricably connected to our overall quality of life. Fortunately, we are at a wonderful place in our history where we can step back, reflect and make bold changes, to become the healthiest versions ourselves possible!

This is why this book offers holistic solutions that work together, to provide a comprehensive approach to wellness. **Circadian360** empowers individuals with both the confidence and abilities to cultivate their own personalized daily practices that will further support the growth and functioning of their mind, body and spirit.

From a 44inch waistline to wearing 32inch-waisted pants today, the most surprising, powerful and inspiring moment thus far in my ongoing wellness journey has been reaching the final boss in this video game of my life, only to realize that I had been fighting myself the whole time. Seriously - the process of living and writing **Circadian360** has been the ultimate reconciliation of self, and I whole-heartedly invite you to experience this actualization.

I want you to experience this because accountability hits you in a different and much more meaningful way, when you're truly walking the walk of the talk that you know you should be speaking and practicing; moreover, when you are divinely moving in your authentic self, after having done any bit of root work to unearth the foundation and sources behind your poor dietary habits, lifestyle choices, perpetual excuses, repeated abusive cycles, etc., you are faced with the choices of either continuing to maintain the existence you once knew (potentially at your own continued detriment and eventual demise) or ascend to a higher and potentially better version of yourself.

Yes - for many of us, **Circadian360** will be the ultimate red pill / blue pill moment in our own living Matrix: a moment when you can either read the book and go back to your old ways of living, or, you can face the truth, accept responsibility, become accountable and then seize yet another opportunity to move forward with grace, to begin living the life you deserve.

This is why I say: **"Upgrade your light, and you'll upgrade your life."**

Through this book, I invite you to reconnect with the inquisitive light and spirit of your youth, remembering when you questioned the brightness of the sun, the blue sky, and the workings of the human body. As you proceed in your ongoing journey towards improved health and wellness, remember the following:

- Have patience with yourself and others – we are all operating with varying skill sets.

- On your path towards becoming, be careful not to backslide into self-destructive behaviors; rather, in those testing moments, challenge yourself to rise and exist as your future self.

- **Not every caterpillar becomes a butterfly**. Due to potential environmental factors, stress, anxiety, diet, lack of preparation, fear and many more reasons, some caterpillars don't go into chrysalis- the hard-shelled pupal stage when an insect undergoes metamorphosis, transforming from a larva (caterpillar) into an adult. How many bright, talented and gifted individuals have each of us known who never seemed to grow their wings and soar? Maybe it was the way that they were raised, their home environment, the people that they kept around them and/or their dietary factors, addictions, struggles…whatever. The point: Some of the best individuals that we may meet and know may never ascend to their highest authentic selves for a multitude of reasons. Either a caterpillar will do the work at all costs to become their butterfly self…or they won't, don't and/or can't. So I encourage you: Do what you must, to transform into the butterfly that you are.

Thank you to the talented artists, editors, typesetters and designers who helped bring this book into fruition; moreover, together, we created the informative images in this book that intentionally represent brown skin individuals! Growing up, I never saw myself represented in books about the human anatomy, and it is truly a proud honor of mine to be able to do so in **Circadian360**.

I could not write this book alone, and I extend humbled gratitude for each individual who has contributed towards the research findings and resources offered in this book.

Special thanks to my ancestors, family (Rodney & Helen-Arnold Massey (parents); Jahmann Y. Massey (brother)), late pioneering herbalist mentors (William "Bill" Brevoort and Kim "Ki'i" Nakamura), Stefan Thomas and The Interledger Foundation (ILF), friends (Zachary Piercy, Gabriel Abbas, Amanda Perez, Samantha Tate, Amber Vaughn-Wainwright, Elizabeth "Biz" Gonik, Christopher & Portia Mathews-Koenig, Justin Lewis, Jeff & Aaron Heagle, Tim & Juliet Laughlin, Laurie Beckstead, Folakemi Omisore, Benjamin J. Landsman, Adam Fons, Ashley Marie Downing, and Brendan Bowser) and the entire MICOPEIA community.

May this book, rooted in ancient wisdom and modern science, serve you and all of our future generations.

Remember: Your health is a treasure; Nurture it, protect it and let your light shine!

-R. A. Massey

Circadian360

Welcome To Circadian360!

We honor ancient and powerful, researched-backed connections in **Circadian360**. It has been said that the circadian rhythm aligns us with all lifeforms on Earth through a profound, cyclical connection to the energy of the sun and the universe.

The Earth's rotation creates a day and night cycle, establishing a consistent pattern of light and darkness. This cycle serves as a fundamental cue for synchronizing biological rhythms across all species on our planet.

Many of us are unaware that the sun's energy, manifested through wavelengths of light, influences the expression of genes and the secretion of hormones that govern our biological processes. Our sun helps regulate sleep-wake patterns, hormone production, metabolism, and other essential functions. This cannot be emphasized enough: aligning our biological rhythms with the sun's energy ensures optimal coordination of physiological processes, promoting health and well-being within the body.

The intricate interplay between the circadian rhythm, the sun's energy, and the universe reflects the profound interconnectedness of life on Earth. It underscores the harmony between us as organisms and our environment, highlighting the profound impact of natural cycles and celestial forces on the health and functioning of all living beings.

Sadly, just as professional athletes lose their expert ability, our circadian rhythm becomes less efficient, both over time and through mismanagement. Studies show that factors such as aging, reduced outdoor sunlight exposure, overuse of electronic devices emitting blue light, and nighttime eating are 'flattening' our circadian rhythm.

When this happens, potential health issues arise, including hypertension, obesity, insulin intolerance, kidney disease, liver damage, reproductive dysfunctions, and neurobehavioral disorders. This is why we must ensure that the alignment of our biological rhythms is in sync with the sun's energy, and the **Circadian360** book is here to help guide and support your efforts in doing so.

What's The Circadian Rhythm, And Why Does It Matter?

The term "circadian" is derived from the Latin words "Circa," meaning "around," and "diem," meaning "day," and the circadian rhythm is one of the biological rhythms that are _crucial_ for regulating our bodily functions, including sleep, temperature control, and even some of our hormonal changes.

This all happens due to the constant dance between our bodies and the sun.

You see, sunlight serves as a vital cue for the brain's internal clock, known as the suprachiasmatic nucleus (SCN), which then determines when these various functions take place in the body.

Just as a solar panel is constructed to harness the light of the sun to output energy, we human beings are also solar-powered and programmed to wake and rest according to the sun; moreover, many of us are entirely unaware that sunlight significantly influences numerous bodily processes, including cardiovascular health, digestion, and even mental health!

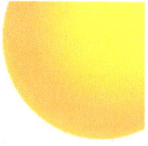

Photoneuroendocrine System

MORNING SUNLIGHT ENSURES PROPER SLEEP

When exposed to morning sunlight in the specified wavelength range (around 450-500nm), the Suprachiasmastic Nucleus (SCN) sends inhibitory signals to the paraventricular nucleus (PVN) of the hypothalamus. The PVN, in turn, helps regulates melatonin release from the pineal gland. Melatonin suppression during the day and its release at night are crucial components of the body's sleep-wake cycle.

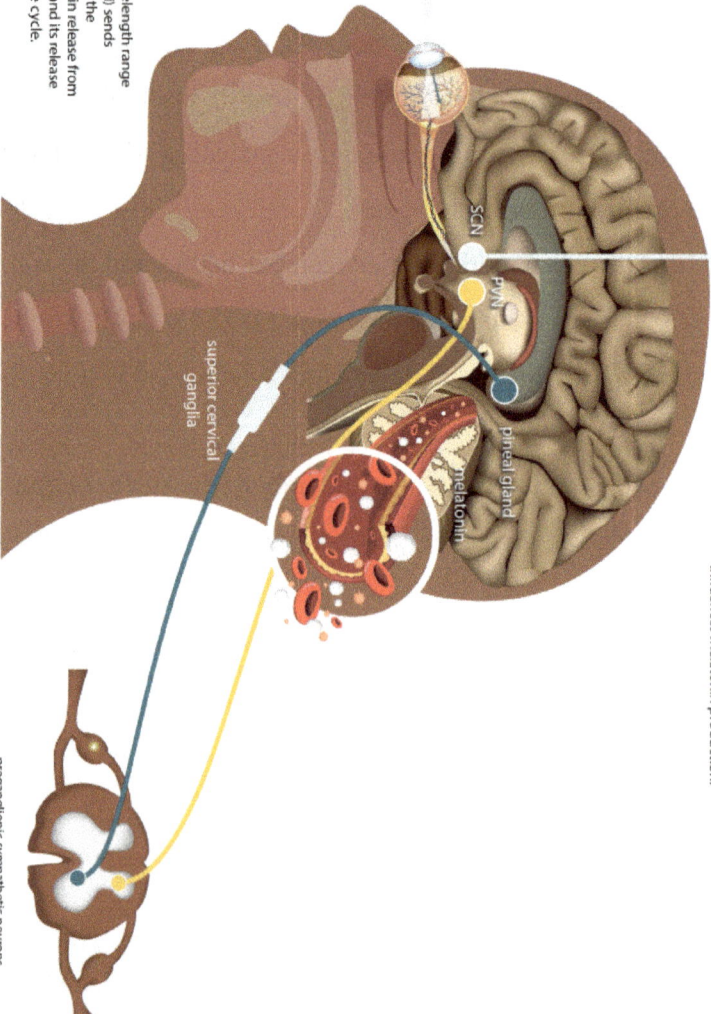

CIRCADIAN360

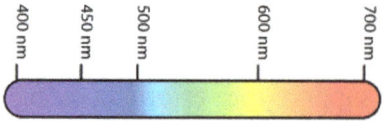

1 Morning sunlight between 450-500nm wavelength is critical for setting circadian rhythm via ganglia cells on the retina.

400 nm
450 nm
500 nm
600 nm
700 nm

2 The suprachiasmatic nucleus (SCN) receives melanopsin signals from retina and passes inhibitory signals on to the preganglionic sympathetic neurons of the spinal cord.

3 When stimulated by the superior cervical ganglion, a part of the sympathetic nervous system, the pineal gland can release norepinephrine, a neurotransmitter and hormone, which influences melatonin production.

SCN
PVN
pineal gland
melatonin
superior cervical ganglia
preganglionic sympathetic neurons

CIRCADIAN360

28

Exposure to bright light, particularly in the morning, has been shown to help regulate our body clocks.

Bright sunlight exposure specifically assists in resetting the SCN, directly impacting the health of our pineal gland. The pineal gland generates melatonin, a hormone tightly linked to our circadian rhythm. This hormone impacts various bodily functions, including blood sugar, cholesterol levels, mental health conditions, immune system functioning, DNA repair, and even the efficacy of cancer treatments.

Melatonin is often called the "sleep hormone" because its levels typically rise in the evening. What's fascinating is that this rise signals to the body that it's time to prepare for sleep. This is why when we spend those long days doing an activity outdoors, whether camping, walking, socializing, etc., we tend to get naturally tired as the sun is setting, whereas exposure to natural light, especially in the morning, suppresses melatonin production. This is part of the body's way of promoting wakefulness during the day. It's why it's so challenging to sleep in after the sun starts beaming on your face—your body is literally AWAKENED by the sun. Similarly, in the evening, as the sunlight dims and has less blue component, melatonin production increases, promoting sleepiness and preparing your body for restorative sleep.

Normally, disruptions to biological rhythms occur due to natural changes in age or environmental factors; however, it seems that since the 3rd Industrial Revolution, more unnatural disruptions have emerged in our world, helping to both give rise to and feed epidemics in cardiovascular disease, metabolic health, cancer, depression, anxiety, insomnia, neurological disorders, immune function, and both genetic and epigenetic concerns. For instance, with the advent of airplanes has come jet lag disorder caused by travel across time zones; moreover, with more demands on the labor economy, we now have an epidemic in shift work disorder stemming from non-traditional work schedules (working 8 to 12 hours or more per shift or overnight hours).

Most alarmingly, with the rise of television, computers, and now Light Emitting Diodes (LEDs), in the span of less than 100 years, we may have paved the foundation for longterm detrimental harm to our health. We are beginning to hear the trickles of voices shouting from new research telling us that artificial blue light is significantly harming us. I imagine the information will be so well known in time that we will evolve into something different; however, the damage to many will have already been done.

Did you know that the blue light you see in the sky due to Rayleigh scattering is related to the blue light emitted by LEDs?

Both types of blue light have a similar appearance because they involve light in the blue part of the visible spectrum. The blue light in the sky is natural sunlight scattered by the Earth's atmosphere, while LED lights are artificial sources containing blue light created using semiconductor technology. LED lights can be much more intense and concentrated compared to the relatively diffuse blue light from the sky, and this intensity does have significant adverse effects on our overall health.

What ends up happening is that the blue light from screens tricks the brain into thinking it's still daytime, suppressing melatonin production and making it more challenging to fall asleep. Even with older tube-style televisions, staring at the TV screen for extended periods late at night contributed to sleep disruptions. Yes - that's why your Mama was saying, "*Don't sit too close to the tv,*" and, "*Don't stay up late watching tv!*" It didn't take a rocket scientist to know that kids were turning into zombies, no longer going outside to play and explore because they were slowly becoming hooked to watching Howdy Doody all damn day. It just took an observant mother. Now, today, contingent on the television program, news broadcast, computer application, website, app, social media platform, texting service, or even your LED nightlights and household lightbulbs, the continual jolts of excitement and stimulation from these artificial light sources are keeping the brain in an awake mode, fully engaged and alert.

So imagine, since the beginning of the 3rd Industrial Revolution, we have been slowly reproducing offspring, descendant generations, to be born into a world lit by artificial lights. For access to this 24/7, 365 consumer casino, you're paying with your finances, your actual time on Earth, and your life-force/Qi/energy.

It is time to upgrade our light to upgrade our life!

Maintaining the synchronization of biological rhythms involves developing unique, signature healthy lifestyle habits and routines rooted in various daily practices, including exposure to sunlight, an established and consistent sleep schedule, daytime physical movement, limiting caffeine consumption and artificial light exposure, and minimizing long naps.

Let me be clear - these routines must become what I call "*Non-Negotiables*" in your life!

Many of us have been born into worlds, communities and households functioning under a preset agreed upon system managed by whatever the authority figure was/is; alarmingly, many of us have never taken the time to separate ourselves from many of our lifestyle habits that were inherited from our ancestors and environments, with an objective and discerning purpose to let go and adopt healthier behaviors and patterns. Now, we are forced to reckon with this heightened awareness granted to our living generations, as it has become crucial for our survival.

As you proceed throughout *The Big Picture* section of this book, you will find that **Circadian360** is navigating you on a journey to learn more about our biological rhythms and the sacred light connection that connects and roots all of us. Through *The Big Picture*, we take a journey that refreshes our understanding of vibrations, frequencies, and the universal needs of all human beings on Earth, highlighting the song of frequencies that harmonize to make our universe. In the section after that, we will utilize our microscope to explore *The Cellular Level* of the human being, highlighting everything from vitamins, minerals, and root causes of illness and disease to comprehensive guides for conducting self-assessments using ancient practices.

Circadian360 offers you a robust collection of tools to establish a strong foundation for self-reliance and accountability in managing your overall health and constitution. From telescope to microscope, this book acknowledges the intricate musicality of vibrations, frequencies, and the power of our choices in making the most of our health and wellness journeys.

May this book serve as a timeless collection of tenets honoring various self-care practices for the human body on Earth.

The Big Picture

Everything in the universe has a vibration and frequency, and YOU are a BEING of LIGHT!

The vibrations and frequencies of the universe, the solar system, and Earth are interconnected, constantly interacting with all life forms on our planet.

Every day, more research-backed evidence is being uncovered supporting the ancient, ancestral belief that the Earth's frequencies and our cosmic clock are connected to our **body clock**.

The **cosmic clock refers to the rhythmic movement of celestial bodies such as the sun, moon, and planets through the cosmos**. Our **body clock**, also known as the **circadian rhythm**, is a natural internal process that regulates our sleep-wake cycle and other bodily functions over a roughly 24-hour period. Our body clock is influenced by external factors such as sunlight and temperature and plays a critical role in maintaining our overall health and well-being. So the rise and fall of the sun and moon, for example, actually signals our bodies to release hormones that help us wake up in the morning and sleep at night.

Science proves that we are light beings with a biological makeup that is inextricably connected and governed by our sun.

Many ancient cultures, including Native American, African, Ayurvedic, and Traditional Chinese Medicine, have long understood and respected our body clock, developing timeless practices that align with the cosmic clock. Our ancestors knew that by following nature's rhythms, we can maintain good health and prevent disease.

Consider this: history has a tendency to repeat itself.

With this, by studying the songs and rhythms of our universe (these naturally occurring vibrations, frequencies, and harmonies), we are both educating ourselves and connecting with the soul of the universe to prepare our future, all while gaining a deeper understanding of the complex systems that make up our world and the universe as it is today.

Fortunately, now is one of the best times to be doing the work to activate your higher self. From 2020 through 2025, we are in a period known as a **Solar Maximum Cycle**.

Solar maximum cycles are periods of heightened solar activity characterized by increased sunspots and solar flares, which are massive energy swells and ejections that come directly from the sun. While solar maximum cycles have been observed for centuries, the understanding and tracking of these cycles have become more accurate recently; moreover, to me, what's fascinating is that these cosmic events have always coincided with MAJOR events, eras and births on Earth.

In the context of **Circadian360**, the Solar Maximum Cycle serves as a profound backdrop, symbolizing not just heightened solar activity, but also a period of spiritual significance and cosmic alignment. During these cycles, the barriers between the physical and metaphysical realms seem to thin, allowing for a deeper connection with the universal energy. It is a time when our potential for spiritual growth and understanding expands, offering us a unique opportunity to attune ourselves to the profound cosmic forces that influence our lives. Through this alignment, we can tap into the transformative power of the universe, embracing our higher selves, and unlocking the mysteries of existence.

Solar Maximum Period	Important Events	Notable Births
1787 - 1798	**French Revolution:** The French Revolution began in 1789, a time of political and social upheaval in France that eventually led to the end of the monarchy.	- Wolfgang Amadeus Mozart (1756-1791): The renowned Austrian composer and musician known for his contributions to classical music was alive during this period. - Mary Shelley (1797-1851): The English novelist best known for her Gothic novel "Frankenstein," was born in 1797.
1809 - 1823	**War of 1812:** A conflict between the United States and Great Britain, the War of 1812 lasted until 1815 and significantly impacted North American history.	- Charles Darwin (1809-1882): The British naturalist and scientist known for his theory of evolution and his book "On the Origin of Species" was born during this period. - Edgar Allan Poe (1809-1849): The American writer and poet renowned for his macabre and Gothic tales was also born during this time.

1837 - 1850	**Industrial Revolution:** The Industrial Revolution, marked by significant advancements in manufacturing, technology, and agriculture, transformed society and the economy.	- Alexander Graham Bell - Born on March 3, 1847. - Claude Monet - Born on November 14, 1840. - Auguste Renoir - Born on February 25, 1841. - Thomas Edison - Born on February 11, 1847.
1859 *(Carrington Event)*	In September 1859, during the peak of this solar maximum cycle, a powerful solar flare and associated coronal mass ejection (CME) occurred. This event is known as the Carrington Event after the astronomer Richard Carrington observed it. It caused widespread disruptions in telegraph systems, resulting in telegraph operators receiving electric shocks and fires starting in some telegraph offices. It is considered one of the most severe solar storms recorded and serves as a reminder of the potential impact of solar activity on modern technological infrastructure.	- Georges Seurat: The French post-Impressionist painter known for his pointillism technique was born on December 2, 1859. - Henri Bergson: The French philosopher and Nobel Prize laureate in Literature was born on October 18, 1859. - Carrie Chapman Catt: The American women's suffrage leader and founder of the League of Women Voters was born on January 9, 1859.
1928 - 1930 - This solar *maximum cycle occurred*	**The Great Depression:** The stock market crash of 1929 marked the	- Maya Angelou: The American poet,

during the early days of radio broadcasting. *The increased solar activity caused significant disruptions to radio communication, leading to the discovery of the relationship between solar activity and radio wave propagation.*	beginning of the Great Depression, a severe worldwide economic downturn throughout the 1930s. It profoundly impacted global economies and societies, leading to high unemployment rates, bank failures, and significant social and political changes.	memoirist, and civil rights activist known for her acclaimed work "I Know Why the Caged Bird Sings" was born on April 4, 1928. - Martin Luther King Jr.: The iconic American civil rights leader and Nobel Peace Prize laureate was born on January 15, 1929. - Anne Frank: The German-born Jewish diarist known for her diary "The Diary of a Young Girl," was born on June 12, 1929. - Andy Warhol: The American artist and leading figure in the visual art movement, known as pop art, was born on August 6, 1928. - Neil Armstrong: The American astronaut who became the first person to walk on the moon was born on August 5, 1930.

1957 - 1958 - This solar maximum cycle coincided with the International Geophysical Year (IGY), a global effort to study various Earth and space sciences aspects. *The increased solar activity during this period provided valuable data for scientists involved in the IGY, contributing to advancements in solar physics and space weather research.*	The **Space Age** Begins: In October 1957, the Soviet Union successfully launched Sputnik 1, the world's first artificial satellite. This event marked the beginning of the Space Age and triggered the space race between the United States and the Soviet Union.	- Michael Jackson: The influential American singer, songwriter, and pop culture icon was born on August 29, 1958.
1989 – 1991- In March 1989, a powerful solar storm caused a geomagnetic storm on Earth during this solar maximum cycle. *The geomagnetic storm resulted in a widespread power outage in the Canadian province of Quebec, affecting millions of people.* *This event highlighted the potential vulnerabilities of power grids to space weather disturbances.*	- **Fall of the Berlin Wall:** In November 1989, the Berlin Wall, which had divided East and West Berlin since 1961, was opened, leading to the eventual reunification of Germany. This event symbolized the end of the Cold War era and significantly impacted European politics and the global geopolitical landscape. - **Gulf War:** The Gulf War, also known as the Persian Gulf War, lasted from 1990 to 1991. It was a military conflict triggered by Iraq's invasion of Kuwait. A coalition of nations led by the United States	- Emma Watson: The British actress, best known for portraying Hermione Granger in the "Harry Potter" film series, was born on April 15, 1990. - Daniel Radcliffe: The British actor, famous for playing the role of Harry Potter in the "Harry Potter" film series, was born on July 23, 1989. - Taylor Swift: The American singer-

<table>
<tr>
<td></td>
<td>intervened to liberate Kuwait from Iraqi occupation. These are just a few examples of the many historical events during the specified years and spans. These events significantly impacted the world and continue to shape our history and collective memory.</td>
<td>songwriter and multiple Grammy Award winner was born on December 13, 1989.</td>
</tr>
</table>

So, if history *is* repeating itself, we will look back at this period of solar maximum potentially as a life-changing era for many in our generation.

On such an affirming note, let us begin our adventure!

You And The Universe Are A Vibe!

Yes - The universe is a big vibe!

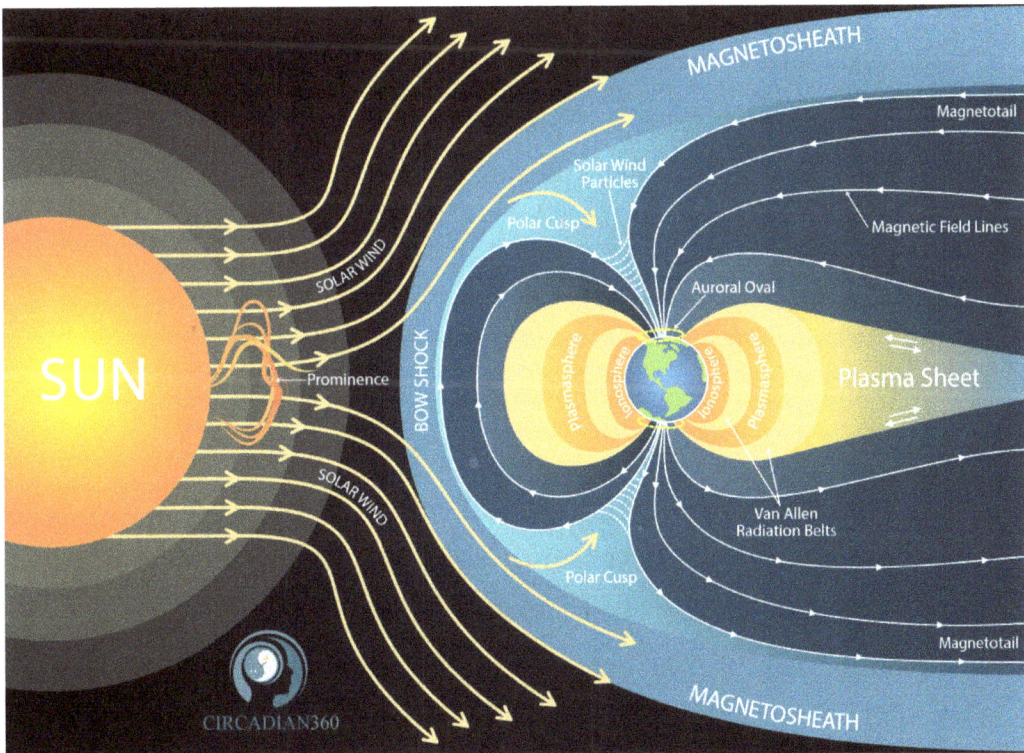

When we look outward to the vastness of space, the Sun shines like a colossal star. It could snugly hold a million Earths inside if you imagined it hollow, with room to spare. Among the stars in the galaxy, it's not the biggest, but its proximity to us sets it apart.

Plasma, a state of matter consisting of charged particles, forms the Sun. These particles dance through magnetic and electric fields, much like the Sun's conversion of its massive core into energy through a process known as nuclear fusion. This process triggers expansive swirling motions akin to the graceful movements of the oceans on Earth. These movements stretch and twirl the Sun's magnetic fields, forming an intricate pattern.

Unlike Earth's steady spin, the middle part of the Sun spins *FASTER* than its top and bottom. Remember those spinning toy tops? Imagine if it spun faster at its center! This causes the Sun's magnetic fields to twist and rise, creating bright spots and loops we see from a distance. It's like a radiant collaboration of light and magnetism.

Just like the universe, the Sun vibrates with a grand sensation. As human beings, our purpose echoes this grandeur as we dance in harmony with the Earth's heartbeat.

The frequency of the universe itself is estimated to be around 432 Hz. This is known as the "universal frequency"; it is believed to have healing and restorative properties for the human body. Some researchers have suggested that many ancient musical instruments, such as the Indian sitar or the Tibetan singing bowl, were tuned to this frequency precisely because of its positive effects on the body.

Moving closer to home, we find that the frequency of the sun, the most prominent celestial body in our solar system, is a staggering 160.2 million Hz. In the form of electromagnetic radiation, this frequency reaches the earth and influences everything from the planet's climate to the growth and development of plants and animals.

When the Sun is active, it emits various forms of energy, including radio waves. The 10.7 cm radio flux is a way to quantify the strength of these radio emissions. The level of radio flux can vary over time, with higher values indicating increased solar activity.

Solar activity is associated with sunspots, solar flares, and coronal mass ejection events that release large amounts of energy and matter from the Sun's surface into space. These events can affect Earth's space environment, including disruptions in radio communications, interference with satellite operations, and changes in Earth's magnetic field. These periods of high solar activity also lead to colorful auroras in the sky. This brings us right back to the start of this section, where we acknowledged the impact of solar maximum cycles as periods of heightened solar activity, and an increased number of sunspots and solar flares characterizes these periods.

It's crucial that we reset our way of being and embrace healthier lifestyles. We must understand that the frequency of the universe, the cosmic clock, the Sun, the Earth, and the human body clock are all intricately connected, influencing and shaping each other in a never-ending dance of vibrations and rhythms. This testament is our birthright, reminding us of the beauty and complexity of the universe and the profound interconnection between all things.

Vibrations Vs. Frequencies

Vibrations and frequencies are closely related, but they are not the same.

Vibrations are physical movements that oscillate back and forth, often disturbing the surrounding medium. This is shown when you pluck a guitar string. It vibrates back and forth, causing the air molecules around it to vibrate. These vibrations in the air produce sound waves, which are perceived by our ears as sound. *Isn't that fascinating?*

On the other hand, frequency refers to the rate at which these vibrations or oscillations occur. Specifically, it refers to the number of oscillations or cycles that occur in one second, measured in Hertz (Hz).

So, in essence, vibrations are the physical movements that create sound waves, while frequency measures the rate at which these movements occur.

However, *what causes these vibrations in the first place?*

There are many different vibration sources, ranging from physical objects to electromagnetic waves.

When you speak, your vocal cords vibrate, producing sound waves that are heard as speech. Similarly, seismic waves traveling through the Earth's crust during an earthquake produce vibrations that seismometers can detect.

In the case of electromagnetic waves, such as those emitted by the sun or other celestial bodies, the vibrations are produced by the movement of charged particles. When these particles move, they create an electromagnetic field that oscillates back and forth, producing energy waves that can travel through space.

All human beings can be said to be made up of vibrations and frequencies, and this is because everything in the universe, including our bodies, is made of atoms, which are made up of subatomic particles such as protons, neutrons, and electrons.

These particles are constantly in motion, producing electromagnetic waves, which can be measured in frequency and wavelength.

Every object, including our bodies, has its own unique frequency or set of frequencies, which can be measured and analyzed using various tools and techniques.

Electroencephalography (EEG) is a technique that measures the brain's electrical activity, which can be analyzed in terms of frequency to determine a person's brainwave pattern; moreover, heart rate variability (HRV) measures the variation in time between successive heartbeats, which can be analyzed in frequency to determine a person's heart rate variability pattern.

So, *it may be* oversimplifying it to say that we are "made up" of vibrations and frequencies; however, our bodies and the things around us are constantly vibrating and oscillating, producing unique patterns of electromagnetic waves that can be measured and analyzed in terms of frequency and wavelength.

Plants have been shown to respond to various vibrations and frequencies, including sound and electromagnetic waves. Yes - studies have shown that plants can grow differently depending on the frequency and intensity of the sound waves they are exposed to.

Two studies that have shown the effect of sound waves on plant growth are the

"Biomusic in Plant Growth" study by Dorothy Retallack in 1973, where she found that plants exposed to classical and jazz music grew towards the source of the music, while those exposed to rock music grew away from it. In the "Effect of Sound Waves on Growth and Physiological Parameters in Plants" study by Singh et al. in 2018, they found that sound waves with a frequency of 20-50 Hz and intensity of 90-95 dB increased the growth rate, leaf area, and chlorophyll content of wheat plants. These studies suggest that sound waves can affect plant growth and may have potential applications in agriculture and horticulture.

As discussed earlier, the universe and our planet have unique vibrations and frequencies, which can be measured and analyzed using various techniques.

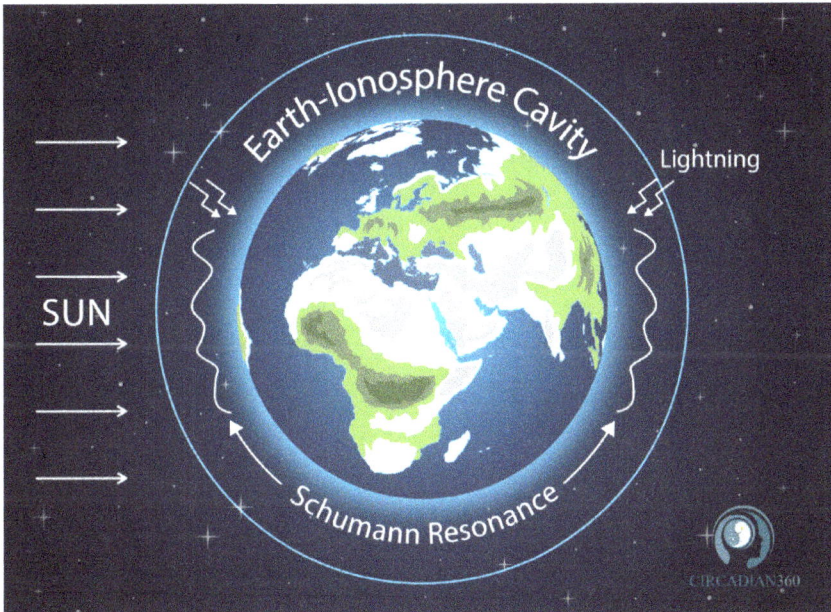

The Schumann Resonances are naturally occurring electromagnetic frequencies between the Earth's surface and the ionosphere. The ionosphere is a region within Earth's upper atmosphere, extending from about 50 miles above the Earth's surface to around 400 miles or more into space. This region is characterized by its high concentration of ions and free electrons, which are charged particles. The ionosphere is formed primarily through the interacting high-energy ultraviolet (UV) and X-ray radiation from the Sun with the neutral gases in the upper atmosphere. Beyond playing a significant role in atmospheric studies, radio signal transmission, and signals from Global Navigation Satellite Systems like GPS satellites, the ionosphere creates auroras, also known as the Northern and Southern Lights. When charged particles from the sun's solar wind interact with the ionosphere's ions and electrons, they emit light, creating colorful displays near the polar regions, distinguishable by visible UV, red and green airglow.

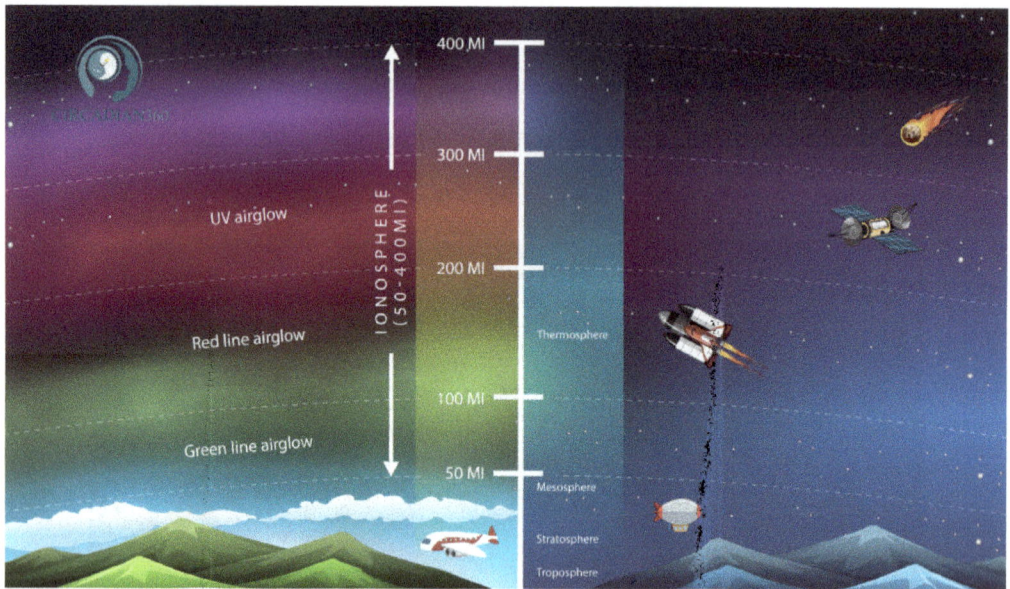

Existing in that space between the Earth's surface and the ionosphere, the Schumann Resonance frequencies are believed to be generated by lightning discharges in the Earth's atmosphere, which create electromagnetic waves that bounce back and forth between the surface and the ionosphere. The primary Schumann Resonance is at a frequency of around 7.83 Hz, but there are other frequencies as well.

Now, giving credit where credit is due, these resonances are named after the German physicist Winfried Otto Schumann, who predicted their existence in 1952. The Schumann Resonances are sometimes called the "heartbeat" of the Earth and are believed to have important implications for the health of living organisms, including humans.

In the 1980s, a study known as the "bunker studies" was conducted by Dr. R.

Becker and Dr. A. Marino. The study isolated individuals from all external electromagnetic frequencies (EMFs) and exposed them only to the Schumann resonance. The researchers found that after a short period, the individuals showed a significant improvement in their depression and other symptoms.

Other studies have examined sound therapy's effects using frequencies similar to the Schumann resonance. One study published in the Journal of Alternative and Complementary Medicine found that sound therapy using a frequency of 7.83 Hz improved heart rate variability and reduced anxiety in participants.

So imagine - the various types of music, entertainment, news broadcasts, media, and environmental sounds you are exposing yourself to impact your present and long-term health.

The Schumann resonance is considered essential for life on Earth, as it is thought to help regulate the body's circadian rhythm and other physiological processes. While natural frequencies such as the Schumann Resonance and sound therapy can positively affect our health, artificial frequencies can have the opposite effect.

With the rise of technology, there has been an increase in electromagnetic frequencies (EMFs) in our environment, such as those emitted from cell phones, Wi-Fi, and other electronic devices. These artificial frequencies can disrupt our body's natural rhythms and cause health problems such as headaches, insomnia, and fatigue.

It is *essential* to be aware of the potential adverse effects of artificial frequencies and take steps to reduce our exposure, such as turning off electronic devices at night and limiting our time spent on screens.

The Energetic Properties Flowing From Water To Food

Water, the elixir of life, holds a fascinating secret: it responds profoundly to frequencies and vibrations, adjusting its molecular structure based on whatever various energetic influences it encounters.

Scientific experiments, notably pioneered by Japanese researcher Dr. Masaru

Emoto, have vividly showcased water's remarkable responsiveness to frequencies. Dr. Emoto's work revealed that positive and negative words, thoughts, and even music have transformative effects on water's crystalline structure under a microscope. The power of intention and emotion was observed to impact the symmetry and beauty of water crystals, underscoring the dynamic relationship between human consciousness and water's molecular arrangement.

Beyond human influence, water molecules resonate with specific frequencies, inducing organizational changes. This resonance acts like a tuning fork, harmonizing with precise frequencies and triggering a cascading effect that influences neighboring water molecules; moreover, natural processes, such as exposure to sunlight, moonlight, and geomagnetic influences, subtly but significantly alter water's molecular arrangement. This intricate interplay between environmental factors and water's inherent properties reveals the fascinating dance within this essential substance.

These revelations not only deepen our understanding of water but also open doors to numerous applications.

In the realm of health and wellness, structured water's potential impact on cellular health is under exploration. In agriculture, structured water may enhance plant growth and nutrient absorption, promising advancements in sustainable farming practices; moreover, technological innovations, including water treatment methods and energy-harvesting devices, could benefit immensely from comprehending water's responsiveness to frequencies.

The dynamic relationship between water and frequencies paints a picture of a living, adaptable substance that harmonizes with its surroundings on a vibrational level. As we dive into the mysteries of water's behavior, we find ourselves on the brink of harnessing its innate potential. From improving human lives to positively shaping the world at large, the possibilities are as boundless as the depths of the oceans themselves.

Consider drinking natural spring water, as it is often hailed as one of the

purest and healthiest choices for hydration, and this preference is rooted in several key factors:

1. Mineral Composition: Natural spring water derives mineral content from the geological formations it passes through. These minerals, including calcium, magnesium, and potassium, contribute to the water's taste and potential health benefits. These minerals can support various bodily functions, from bone health to electrolyte balance.

2. Purity and Source: Spring water typically originates from underground sources protected from pollution and contaminants by layers of rock and soil. This natural filtration process can result in water that is exceptionally pure and free from many of the pollutants found in other water sources.

3. Untouched by Humans: Natural spring water is often sourced directly from underground aquifers, avoiding the need for extensive human processing or treatment. This means it is less likely to have additives like chlorine or fluoride commonly found in tap water.

4. Neutral pH: Many natural spring waters have a naturally balanced pH level, which can promote a healthy balance in the body. A neutral pH can also enhance the water's taste.

5. Potential Health Benefits: While more research is needed, some studies suggest that the minerals present in natural spring water could offer health benefits; for example, magnesium in spring water might contribute to cardiovascular health and reduce the risk of certain chronic diseases.

6. Connection to Nature: Drinking natural spring water can evoke a sense of connection to the Earth and its natural processes. This can enhance the overall sensory experience of drinking water and contribute to a feeling of well-being.

7. Sustainability: Many natural springs provide a renewable source of water that is replenished by rainfall and natural underground flows. Utilizing these sustainable sources can have a lower environmental impact than tapping into groundwater reservoirs.

Fun fact: There are available maps of the United States of America showing exactly where FREE, public, and accessible spring water sources are!

It's important to note that not all natural spring waters are the same, and the quality can vary depending on the source and location. Before drinking, ensure that the spring water is sourced from a reputable and certified source and provider and meets regulatory standards for safety and quality.

Watering Our Relationship With Food

Our relationship with food has been intimately tied to gardening and farming practices since the beginning of human civilization.

Based on history as we know it today, our earliest ancestors were hunters and gatherers who foraged for food; however, the Neolithic period, also known as the New Stone Age, marked a significant transition in human history when societies shifted from a nomadic hunter-gatherer lifestyle to settled agricultural communities. This transition profoundly impacted various aspects of human life, including the development of farming, herbalism, and our relationship with food.

During the Neolithic period, humans began to domesticate plants and animals, leading to the establishment of agriculture. Cultivating crops such as wheat, barley, rice, corn, and others provided a more reliable and abundant food supply than relying solely on hunting and gathering. This shift from a nomadic lifestyle to settled farming communities allowed permanent settlements, population growth, and more complex social structures.

As humans settled into agricultural communities, they more intentionally observed and interacted with the local flora. They discovered the various uses and properties of different plants, leading to the emergence of herbalism. Herbalism involves studying and using plants for medicinal, culinary, and ritual purposes. People learned to identify medicinal plants and developed knowledge about their therapeutic properties, using them to treat ailments and enhance well-being. Herbalism played a vital role in ancient cultures, and many traditional healing practices and systems of medicine, such as African, Ayurveda, and Traditional Chinese Medicine, have deep roots in this period.

A further extension of herbalism, the shift to agriculture during the Neolithic period, brought about a fundamental change in the human relationship with food. Instead of relying on various wild food sources available through hunting and gathering, people began cultivating specific crops and domesticating animals for food production. This development in food production allowed for increased control over the food supply and the ability to sustain larger populations. It also led to the development of culinary traditions, food processing techniques, and the preservation of surplus food for storage. As communities became more settled, the cultivation of specific crops and the domestication of animals became deeply ingrained in their cultures, shaping dietary patterns and culinary practices that have persisted through the ages.

The Neolithic period was a pivotal time in human history.

The transition to farming, the exploration of herbalism, and the transformation of our relationship with food laid the foundation for the development of civilizations and the shaping of our modern societies. The practices and knowledge that emerged during this period continue to influence agriculture, medicine, and our understanding of the vital connection between humans and the natural world. In time, the ancient Sumerians, Egyptians, and Greeks would all have advanced farming practices, even building gardens, like the Hanging Gardens of Babylon, considered one of the Seven Wonders of the World.

Sadly, with the advent of the 3rd Industrial Revolution, how we grew and consumed food drastically changed.

Technological advances allowed for mass food production and the rise of processed and fast foods, leading to a decline in our consumption of fresh, whole foods. This shift in dietary habits has contributed to the rise of chronic diseases, such as obesity, diabetes, and heart disease. In fact, the World Health Organization estimates that approximately 80% of premature heart disease, stroke, and type 2 diabetes cases can be prevented by making lifestyle changes, including adopting a healthier diet.

Despite our changes in our food production and consumption habits, the connection between the Earth's vibrations and frequencies, moon cycles, and sun cycles on gardening and farming practices remains unchanged, with research continuing to show their interconnectedness.

The South Korean National Institute of Agricultural Biotechnology found that exposing rice seeds to high-frequency sound waves increased their germination rates and yields; moreover, a study conducted by the University of Florence in Italy found that exposing tomato plants to music, specifically classical and jazz, increased their growth and resistance to disease.

The significance of these findings continues to build upon the foundations of our traditional farming practices. The Farmer's Almanac, for instance, has been around for over 200 years, serving as a guide for farmers and gardeners to optimize their planting and harvesting cycles based on the moon and sun cycles. Our ancestors were aware of the importance of the Earth's vibrational and electromagnetic fields on plant growth, which is why they developed these practices that are still relevant today.

We also now know that the actual acts of gardening and farming benefit our physical, mental and emotional well-being.

A growing body of research supports the notion that spending time in nature and engaging in gardening activities can positively affect mental health. One study published in the Journal of Health Psychology found that just 30 minutes of gardening can significantly reduce levels of the stress hormone cortisol, leading to improved mood and reduced feelings of tension and fatigue. Another study published in the International Journal of Environmental Research and Public Health found that gardening can improve symptoms of depression and anxiety, increase feelings of calmness and relaxation, and promote a sense of connection to the natural world. These findings suggest that incorporating both more time in nature and gardening into our daily lives can significantly benefit mental health.

Grounding or **earthing** refers to connecting oneself with the Earth's energy and establishing a harmonious relationship between our frequency and the Earth's frequency. It involves physically, mentally, and energetically aligning with the Earth's electromagnetic field to promote stability, balance, and well-being. Our relationship with gardening and farming can play a significant role in strengthening this connection.

This is going to surprise many, but we establish a direct physical connection with the Earth's surface through activities like walking barefoot on the ground, working with soil, or planting and tending to plants. This physical contact allows for the transfer of electrons between our bodies and the Earth, which is believed to have grounding effects. This transfer of electrons is facilitated by the conductivity of the Earth's surface and can help balance and stabilize our body's electrical energy. With the Schumann resonance being measured at approximately 7.83 Hz and associated with a state of balance and well-being, gardening and farming also allow us to immerse ourselves in environments where this frequency is naturally present. By spending time in these environments, we can align our energetic frequencies with the Earth's resonance, harmonizing and balancing our overall energy.

So, while some individuals may understand the importance of aligning their crops with the moon and sun cycles, many are still disconnected from this knowledge and its relation to their bodies. Even those who grow their food may lack the understanding of how their body clock works and how it is intricately connected to the cycles of nature. Despite their commitment to healthy and sustainable food practices, farmers and gardeners face health concerns like inflammation, diabetes, and autoimmune disorders. This highlights the need for a deeper understanding of our body clock, its impact on our health, and the importance of aligning our daily habits with the natural rhythms of the world around us.

Elevate Your Energy With High-Frequency Foods, Behaviors, Choices, Clothing & Fragrances

There are those who radiate vitality and positive energy to the point that it is almost as if they have an inner glow that captivates everyone around them. On the other hand, we've all encountered Energy Vampires—individuals whose negative energy drains our vitality.

Everything in the universe, including ourselves, possesses an energetic vibration. Our bodies are not merely a collection of chemical parts but rather intricate systems that operate in harmony with the electromagnetic energy of the universe. This energy can be measured and influenced.

The great inventor Nikola Tesla once said, 'If you want to find the secrets of the universe, think in terms of energy, frequency, and vibration.' This statement holds profound truth.

You, me, and everything around us are essentially bundles of energy vibrating at different frequencies. According to the laws of thermodynamics, energy cannot be created or destroyed; it can only be transferred or transformed. This means we constantly interact with and are influenced by the energy within and around us.

A Healthy Body's Vibrational Frequency

Bruce Tainio was known for his work in bioelectromagnetics and alternative health. He developed the Tainio Technology BFA (Biofield Frequency Analyzer), a device that he claimed could measure the frequencies of living organisms, including the human body.

According to Tainio's assertions, a healthy human body would resonate within a specific frequency range, typically cited as 62-78 MHz (megahertz). This range was said to represent a state of optimal health and well-being. Tainio also claimed that when the body's frequency dropped below a certain threshold, often cited as 58 MHz, it could be more susceptible to diseases.

When the body's frequency falls due to physiological, emotional, or environmental factors, it causes the immune system to become weak, making the body more susceptible to viruses and harmful bacteria.

Based on Tainio's research, here are some frequencies associated with the human body:

- Genius Brain: 80-82 MHz
- Normal Human Body: 62-78 MHz
- Human Colds and Flu start at 57-60 MHz
- The disease starts at 58 MHz
- Candida overgrowth starts at 55 MHz
- Receptive to Cancer at 42 MHz
- Death begins at 25 MHz

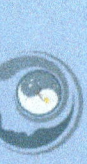

Circadian360's
High Frequency Food Pyramid

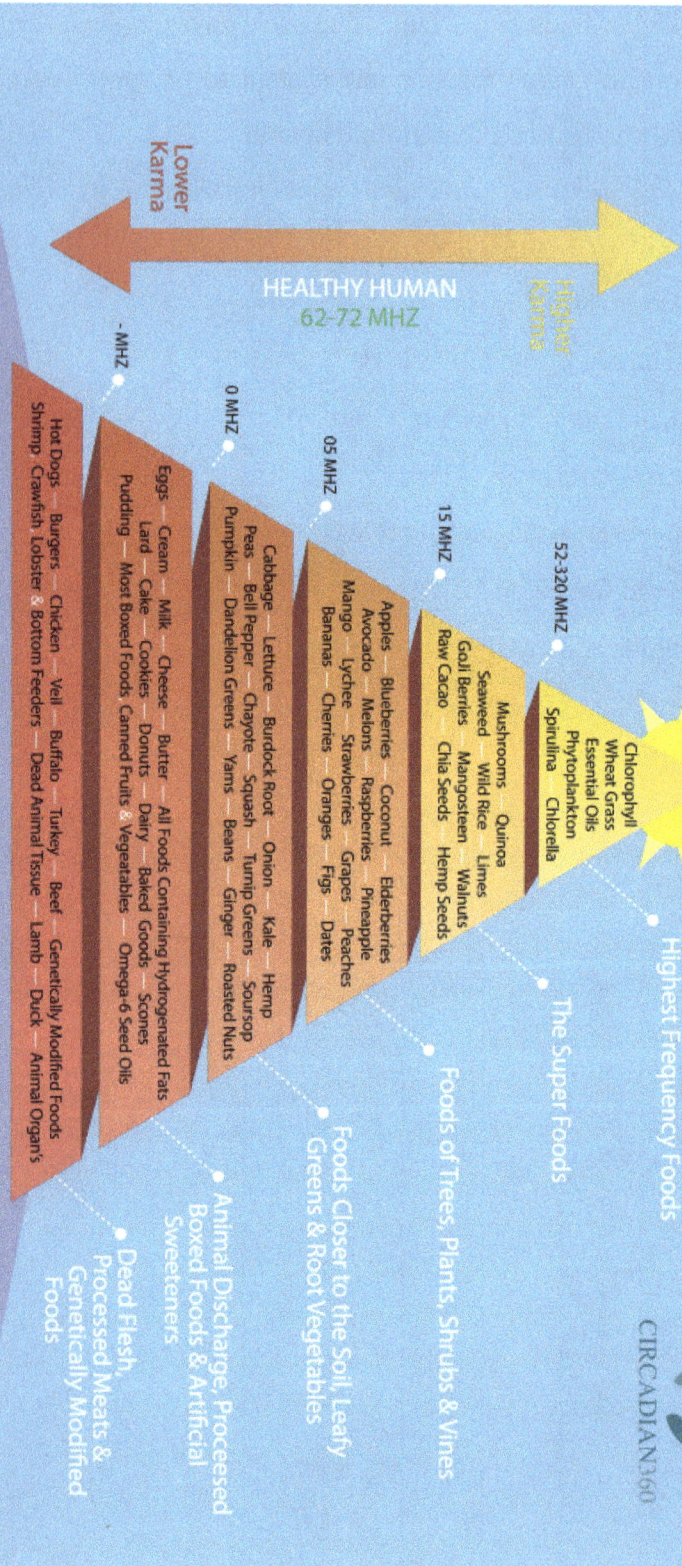

CIRCADIAN360

Lower Karma

Higher Karma

HEALTHY HUMAN
62-72 MHZ

- MHZ

0 MHZ

05 MHZ

15 MHZ

52-320 MHZ

Chlorophyll — Wheat Grass — Essential Oils — Phytoplankton — Spirulina — Chlorella

Mushrooms — Quinoa — Seaweed — Wild Rice — Limes — Goji Berries — Mangosteen — Walnuts — Raw Cacao — Chia Seeds — Hemp Seeds

Apples — Blueberries — Coconut — Elderberries — Avocado — Melons — Raspberries — Pineapple — Mango — Lychee — Strawberries — Grapes — Peaches — Bananas — Cherries — Oranges — Figs — Dates

Cabbage — Lettuce — Burdock Root — Onion — Kale — Hemp — Peas — Bell Pepper — Chayote — Squash — Turnip Greens — Soursop — Pumpkin — Dandelion Greens — Yams — Beans — Ginger — Roasted Nuts

Eggs — Cream — Milk — Cheese — Butter — All Foods Containing Hydrogenated Fats — Lard — Cake — Cookies — Donuts — Dairy — Baked Goods — Scones — Pudding — Most Boxed Foods, Canned Fruits & Vegetables — Omega-6 Seed Oils

Hot Dogs — Burgers — Chicken — Veil — Buffalo — Turkey — Beef — Genetically Modified Foods — Shrimp · Crawfish Lobster & Bottom Feeders — Dead Animal Tissue — Lamb — Duck — Animal Organs

Highest Frequency Foods

The Super Foods

Foods of Trees, Plants, Shrubs & Vines

Foods Closer to the Soil, Leafy Greens & Root Vegetables

Animal Discharge, Proceesed Boxed Foods & Artificial Sweeteners

Dead Flesh, Processed Meats & Genetically Modified Foods

Exploring High-Frequency Foods

Foods in their natural, unprocessed state maintain the highest frequencies. Prioritize growing your own produce and/or buying fresh produce several times a week from local farmer's markets, as supporting local farmers may offer fresher produce compared to supermarket offerings. Store fruits and vegetables in cool, dark, and dry areas to preserve their freshness. If you have land to spare, consider looking into root cellaring.

The vibrational frequency of food also plays a role in our overall well-being. While it's important to note that precise frequencies for individual food items may vary depending on factors such as ripeness, freshness, and quality, the **Circadian360 High Frequency Food Pyramid** offers some general ranges.

Here are different categories of food items based on their vibrational frequency:

Category 1: High-Quality Foods (listed in descending order):
- Sun-ripened fruits or cold-pressed, freshly squeezed fruit juices
- Raw, uncut, non-refrigerated, freshly plucked vegetables
- Sprouts
- Hazelnuts, peanuts, sunflower seeds, coconut, sweet almonds, olives
- Legumes
- Herbs, spices
- Fermented foods
- Herbal teas (non-caffeinated)

Category 2 – Medium-Quality Foods:
- Lightly cooked fresh vegetables
- Cold-pressed peanut oil
- Raw honey
- Raw cacao

- Sugar cane and wine

Category 3 – Low-Quality Foods (listed in descending order):
- Coffee and caffeinated teas
- Chocolates
- Pickles, preserves, and jams
- Deep-fried food
- White bread
- Cheese
- Pizza
- Eggs

Category 4 – Foods that Decrease Vibrational Frequency

These foods are incredibly detrimental and have a profoundly negative impact on your energy. They can be described as lifeless and devoid of vitality. Consuming them counteracts all of the positive energy work you're putting in to yourself. Even occasional consumption of these 13 foods are strongly discouraged by other health advocates.

1. Margarine and lard
2. Pasteurized milk
3. Cooked sausages and meats
4. Alcoholic drinks
5. Refined sugar
6. Bleached flour
7. Genetically modified foods
8. Processed foods
9. Ready-to-eat meals like frozen pizzas, soups, etc.
10. Canned vegetables and fruits
11. Foods that contain preservatives and artificial colors

12. All food items containing hydrogenated fats (steer clear of packaged, ready-to-eat foods with extended shelf life)

13. Canned Foods - be careful with your consumption of canned fruits, vegetables, broth and soups! The high sodium will feed inflammation, increase blood pressure and costs you more energy to digest than it is giving you. Also - always rinse off your canned beans!

Feeling Alive with Raw Foods

Consuming fresh, raw foods allows us to mirror nature, showing up in our lives with a thriving, vibrant life force. Remember when they used to say: "You are what you eat?" Well, we are finding through more and more research that this is absolutely true; moreover, the energy, frequency, trauma, diseases, illness, hormonal supplements and other harmful agents that can permeate food sources are certainly passed to us upon consumption.

The notion that we should be abusive to animals, farming them and/or killing them to the point of extinction, while genetically altering their DNA and stripping them of any humane form of life, simply because the Bible states in several passages that God instructed individuals to consume meat for nourishment and sustenance are completely not acknowledging the compassionate dominion by which Biblical figures such as Noah was praised for. How could Noah and his family possibly save every sent animal pair from extinction, then watch them multiply and repopulate life on Earth, if they were determined to abuse God's guidance in consuming meat and herbs of the Earth? The first book of the Bible, Genesis, speaks of the amazing blessing that comes from tending to your own garden, home and being fruitful…and yet, many individuals in our current Western world have no idea where their food came from, let alone the energy, ingredients, practices and intentional frequencies by which their food was raised, harvested and preserved with. In sacrificing our responsibility for convenience, we are now seeing how our own lifestyle choices have shortened both our own lifespans and overall quality of life.

In reconnecting to our food sources, we must recognize that we assimilate the vibrancy and vitality of the foods that we consume, greatly contributing towards our constant journey towards becoming the healthiest versions of ourselves. The longer a food is separated from its birth source, the lower its frequency. Thus, the highest vibrational frequency foods are always organically grown fresh fruits and vegetables from your garden or local farmer's market.

Remember – You ARE what you eat.

Raw foods with juices replenish our body fluids, radiating an undeniable glow in our physical and energetic bodies. Prioritize living, raw foods.

Preserving the Vibrancy of Food by Avoiding Overcooking

As soon as fruits and vegetables undergo any form of processing, they begin losing their electromagnetic charge. If you're in the habit of boiling vegetables under the impression that it's a healthy choice- stop immediately! You are essentially consuming lifeless food devoid of nutritional and energetic value.

If cooking is necessary, lightly steaming vegetables or stir-frying them with a small amount of organic vegetable oil is ideal. Avoid cooking vegetables to the point where their color changes, as even this cooking method diminishes their potency.

It is best to consume fruits in their raw state, as ripe and juicy fruits hold the highest frequency, having been naturally "cooked" by the sun.

Be careful to steer clear of consuming too many fruit juices and smoothies, even if they are certified organic and/or homegrown raw produce. This is because juicing and blending your produce destroys and alters their natural fiber-rich composition. The human body requires both soluble and insoluble fibers to digest foods. When you eat vegetables in their whole form, the fiber helps to create a gooey-like mesh along your gastrointestinal tract. This protective layer then becomes a crucial layer of support, in helping regulate the body's absorption of sugars from food. This is significant, as it helps to reduce the chances of spikes in blood sugar and insulin levels.

Also - be cautious with your consumption of canned fruits, vegetables, broth and soups! The high sodium will feed inflammation, increase blood pressure and costs you more energy to digest than it is giving you. Also - always rinse off your canned beans!

Embracing High-Frequency Individuals

High frequency individuals tend to be magnetic and charming, drawing others towards them. These individuals are not necessarily attractive in conventional ways, but seem to go about life with an irresistible aura around them. High frequency individuals may be described as happy, joyful and always wearing a smile. These folk radiate and glow, both inside and out, with a selfless sense of love, compassion, and kindness.

On the other hand, individuals with a low frequency repel others, and their energy makes people want to avoid them. These individuals have a sometimes sunken, dull and lifeless appearance, lacking vibrancy. Low frequency individuals consume low frequency food and lifestyle habits that result in poor physical health, while being susceptible to various illnesses. These low frequency individuals HABITUALLY make unhealthy lifestyle choices, while maintaining a victim mindset. These individuals don't seek and/or cannot be held accountable for their own choices, potentially seeing themselves as powerless. These individuals utilize the access to information granted through harmful LED technology, as a means to spend their days gazing at television, computer and phone screens, while absorbing a continued barrage of low frequency content. These individuals may engage in low vibrational activities like consuming negative news and/or gossiping, with a habit of criticizing others.

Don't be afraid to reassess certain relationships and environments in your life. If they don't raise your frequency, they are likely draining you, lowering your frequency and/or keeping you stuck so that they don't have to face their own growth journey.

Altering Your Vibrational Frequency

The beauty of energetic vibrations is that they can be altered. Even if you resonate more with the signs of a lower vibrational frequency, you don't have to remain stuck there. You can change and elevate your frequency by making a few lifestyle adjustments.

Thus far, throughout *The Big Picture,* we have explored the understanding that at the core of our existence is within a profound connection to the universe, where we are not only physical beings but also beings of light. The dance of our circadian rhythm, intricately linked to the sun's cycles, illuminates this truth. Just as the sun emits light, we, too, emit energy and vibrations, like frequencies in motion. This understanding leads us to explore the fascinating realm of **epigenetics**, which reveals that our inherited DNA does not solely determine our genetic expression.

Epigenetics teaches us that our lifestyle choices, experiences, and environment can influence how our genes are expressed, fundamentally shaping who we are. It is a profound realization that we can activate or deactivate specific genes through our daily choices and habits.

Epigenetics is like a set of instructions telling your genes when to turn on or off, like a light switch. Our genes are like a blueprint that determines how our bodies work and develop, but epigenetics can add an extra layer of control. Things like our environment, lifestyle choices, and experiences can influence it.

Imagine you have a book with lots of pages. Each page has a different chapter or instruction for your body. Epigenetics is like bookmarks or sticky notes that can be placed on some pages to tell your body which chapters to read or skip. These bookmarks can be influenced by different things around you, like what you eat, how active you are, or even how much you sleep.

Sometimes, these bookmarks can be temporary, like a post-it note that can be easily removed. Other times, they can be more long-lasting, like a permanent marker. These bookmarks can affect how your body functions and responds to its environment. They can even be passed down from parents to children, which is why some traits or conditions can run in families. Oftentimes, this is what we are really trying to achieve when we say we want to 'break generational curses'.

Understanding epigenetics can empower you to make choices that positively influence not only your genes but also your body's internal clock/circadian rhythm. Adopting healthy habits like getting enough sleep, eating nutritious food, and managing stress can positively impact your genes' behavior and overall well-being.

Remember, epigenetics shows us that we have some control over how our genes are expressed.

Our choices and actions can make a difference in our health and development. It's like having a say in how your body's story unfolds, empowering you to shape a healthier, more vibrant future through mindful lifestyle habits. Through taking control of these choices, you are also building the frontal lobe of your brain, improving your social interactions, ability to focus, moral judgements, self-control, positive decision-making, fairness and overall character.

Here are key steps to increase your vibrational frequency and support epigenetic well-being:

1. Diet: Incorporate high-frequency foods and eliminate low-frequency ones to nurture a healthy lifestyle.

2. Exercise: Engage in activities that absorb energetic vibrations, such as tai chi, yoga and dance, while promoting physical well-being.

3. Positive Thoughts and Mindfulness: Surround yourself with positivity, positive people, and uplifting content. Cultivate mindfulness and gratitude, avoiding negative influences. This is why Circadian360 offers the companion Mindfulness &

Manifestations Workbook, to provide tools to support comprehensive healing and wellness.

4. Meditation: Adopt a meditation practice that resonates with you, quickly elevating your energy and enhancing your emotional well-being.

5. Love and Kindness: Embrace a heart-centered approach, sending blessings and loving vibrations to everyone you encounter, fostering positive social connections.

6. Nature and Environmental Awareness: Spend time in nature, particularly at sunrise and sunset, which tend to have higher frequencies. Be aware of environmental factors and reduce exposure to toxins, creating a clean and healthy living environment.

7. Stress Reduction: Incorporate stress-reducing practices such as deep breathing exercises, engaging in hobbies, and finding joy and relaxation in activities.

8. Supportive Social Connections: Foster a sense of community and build positive relationships, influencing epigenetic processes and contributing to overall well-being.

Frequencies of Clothing

Did you know that if you have sheets of linen, they are considered holy attire?

For those familiar with The Bible, the scripture reads: "Thou shalt not wear a garment of divers sorts, *as* of woolen and linen together." Deuteronomy 22:11. In this biblical passage, the prohibition against wearing garments made of diverse fabrics, such as wool and linen combined, is stated.

But what does this mean?

Thanks to modern science, we have learned that fabrics have frequencies and vibrations, and that verse from The Bible is alerting readers to the fact that linen and wool have opposing frequencies that cancel each other out!

WHAT?!

Dr. Heidi Yellen, a respected researcher in the field of fabric science, conducted a comprehensive study on fabrics. Her findings were remarkable, and the conclusion reads as follows:

"The [healthy, aligned] human body has a signature frequency of 100, and organic cotton is 100; therefore, you don't want to wear a garment under 100 that is lower than the frequency of the human body. A sickly, nearly dead person has a frequency of 15, and materials such as polyester, rayon, silk, and spandex register at 15. Science PROVES that any fabric worn that has a frequency of less than 100 puts a strain on us, which causes disease, inflammation, and other sicknesses. The ONLY super fabrics are wool and linen, both measuring in at 5000, which ENERGIZES the body and helps fight disease, but when mixed together, the frequencies cancel each other out and fall to zero. Even wearing a wool sweater on top of a linen outfit in a study collapsed the electric field. The reason for this could be that the energy field of wool flows from left to right while that of linen flows in the opposite direction from right to left."

Fabric, just like everything else, has its vibrational frequency.

As electric light beings, every cell in our body functions as a battery, and the frequency of the fabric we come into contact with can influence us. The vibrational frequency of fabric can affect our energy levels and overall functionality. Linen, crafted from flax, stands out as a natural fabric renowned for its breathability, comfort, and ability to enhance our energetic balance and overall well-being.

Now, let's explore the range of frequency for different fabrics:

1) Super Fabrics: These fabrics have high frequencies that promote healing and maintain health. Linen, made from flax, has a frequency of 5000 MHz. Wool also shares this frequency. Remember - wearing these fabrics separately is important, as mixing them cancels their healing effects.

There is another Super Fabric on the horizon - hemp clothing. Hemp possesses remarkable properties and is likely to become a significant player in the fabric industry. More about hemp and its wonders will be discussed shortly.

2) Healthier Fabrics: Organic cotton falls within a frequency range of 70 to 110 MHz, while non-organic cotton that has been bleached or dyed ranges from 40 to 70 MHz. It is worth noting that certain articles suggest cotton can have even higher signature frequencies, potentially reaching up to 400 MHz.

3) Low Energy Fabrics: Most synthetic fabrics fall into this category, with frequencies below 15 MHz. Rayon, polyester, spandex, Lycra, elastane, nylon, and silk belong here. Although Silk is often associated with luxury, it has a frequency similar to that of a sickly, nearly-dead individual. Wearing low-energy fabrics can strain the body, leading to inflammation, illness, and even emotional issues.

Hemp fabric, in particular, deserves special attention. Renowned researcher Dr. Masaru Emoto suggested that planting hemp in contaminated areas, such as Fukushima, could help purify the environment due to its high vibration.

Hemp offers numerous advantages:

- It has an extremely high vibration.
- It is at least four times stronger than cotton and does not deteriorate after multiple washes.
- It breathes better, preventing odor.
- It retains color better than other natural fabrics.
- It is the strongest thread and can be used for making ropes.
- It naturally filters UV light, offering protection for the skin.
- It nourishes and pampers the skin, promoting overall health.
- It is rich in vitamins and can be used as food for humans and livestock.
- It resists bacterial growth.
- It has various industrial applications, including building foundations with hemp bricks.
- It is water-resistant and fire-resistant.
- It helps regulate body and home temperatures, providing warmth when it's cold and cooling when it's hot.

It's important to note that the vibrational frequency of clothing extends beyond just fabric. Jewelry and eyeglasses also possess their frequencies. There is a growing interest in energy-healing jewelry; chemical dyes in clothing can harm our well-being.

Clothing made from carefully combined synthetic and natural materials, created without harmful chemical dyes, can be biocompatible and positively influence the immune system. On the contrary, poorly made clothing, laden with toxins, can weaken the immune system, contributing to inflammation, allergies, and chronic conditions.

We can enhance our well-being and vitality by choosing fabrics with higher frequencies, like linen, wool, and potentially hemp.

I often observe the growing culture of shoe collectors, thriving and passing down through generations. It strikes me that individuals are investing in what essentially act as artificial Earth Frequency Blockers. It would be perfectly acceptable if the collector understood that these novel frequency blockers should not replace spending time barefoot on the Earth to ground the body's frequency with the Earth; however, these uninformed actions perpetuates a cycle of consumerism that often disregards the crucial understanding of how these choices impact our overall well-being, leaving many uninformed and affected.

Let us embrace the profound impact that fabric vibrations can have on our health. I invite you to make conscious choices, opting for fabrics like linen, wool, or hemp, and consider spending more time barefoot on the Earth to ground your body's frequency. By doing so, we nurture ourselves in the most natural and harmonious way.

Frequencies of Essential Oils

We already know that there is a science to formulating perfumes, colognes, and fragrances; nevertheless, did you know that they also may hold vibrations?

In some ways, the vibrational frequency of therapeutic-grade essential oils surpasses all other healing frequencies known to humanity, ranging from 52 to 320

MHz. Essential oils can shape your environment into an inhospitable realm for disease-causing bacteria, viruses, and fungi. So here, quality matters. Lower-grade oils possess lower vibrational levels that can negatively impact you; moreover, allergies associated with essential oil usage often stem from these inferior oils.

When you breathe in these aromatic wonders, their captivating scents travel through the olfactory nerve cells, reaching the brain. Once there, they reach the limbic system—a powerhouse responsible for memory, emotions, and stimulation/arousal. This is why certain smells and fragrances can transport you back to a memory long forgotten; moreover, you can experience heightened alertness or deep relaxation depending on the oil used..

Now, here's the fascinating part. When you apply essential oil directly to your skin, the body rapidly absorbs its antioxidant properties. As a result, you experience a boost in your immunity, a lift in your mood, and a surge of energizing vitality. It's like a revitalizing elixir for your whole being!

These oils possess the power to cleanse cell-surface receptors, making citrus essential oils a top recommendation for this purpose. They can even aid in rewriting faulty DNA programming, offering a beacon of hope in the realm of cancers and autoimmune diseases.

But that's not all! Essential oils have the ability to reprogram DNA and RNA to combat bacterial pathogens, fungi, and disease-causing microbes (cinnamon, clove, and oregano oils are particularly potent here). They enhance the body's natural healing and restorative abilities while relieving depression, dementia, and mood disorders. Depending on the chosen oil, they can induce relaxation and alertness, boosting happiness and overall well-being.

Now, let's talk about the crème de la crème—the essential oils with the highest vibrational frequency!!

Let's revisit the discoveries of esteemed researcher Bruce Tainio, who dedicated his efforts to uncovering the secrets of vibrational frequency. His extensive research revealed that therapeutic-grade pure rose oil leads the pack with an astonishing frequency of 320 MHz. Helichrysum follows suit at 181 MHz, and lavender takes third place at a respectable 118 MHz. These oils reign supreme in the realm of vibrational frequency.

Tainio's experiments even ventured into the realm of thoughts—negative thoughts were found to lower the frequency of essential oils by a staggering 12 MHz; however, when these oils were exposed to positive thoughts, their frequency soared, increasing by 10 MHz.

…and brace yourself for this revelation: Prayer had the most profound effect, elevating the oils' frequency by 15 Hz.

<u>Here are frequencies associated with other popular oils:</u>
Peppermint Essential Oil: 78 MHz
Myrrh Essential Oil: 105 MHz
Lavender Essential Oil: 118 MHz
Frankincense Essential Oil: 147 MHz
Helichrysum Essential Oil: 181 MHz
Rose Essential Oil: 320 MHz

The Vibrant World Of Gemstones: Frequencies, Cultural Traditions, And Holistic Health

In a world where spiritual energies and electromagnetic frequencies profoundly influence our lives, gemstones are fascinating entities with unique vibrations. Throughout history, cultures like the ancient Egyptians and Chinese recognized the intrinsic power of crystals and gemstones. Egyptians used lapis lazuli for spiritual enlightenment, while the Chinese valued jade for its protective properties, employing them for healing, technological advancements, and overall well-being.

In this section, we'll highlight the scientific properties and spiritual significance of gemstone frequencies. We'll also explore how different cultures have integrated gemstones into their healing practices.

Gemstone Frequencies

Gemstones are not merely inert objects. They possess distinct molecular structures that emit subtle vibrations. These vibrations, often referred to as frequencies, interact with the subtle energy fields surrounding living organisms, influencing physical, emotional, and spiritual states. This concept resonates with the principles of energy medicine, which suggest that each gemstone emits a unique frequency that can impact our bioenergetic systems.

Crystals possess extraordinary power beyond our current understanding, and science has only begun to unravel the secrets hidden within their intricate structures.

In a 1964 video by the United States Air Force, viewers were introduced to how crystals are utilized in oscillator circuits. These circuits generate stable frequencies, a crucial factor in preventing interference between radio stations operating on nearby frequencies. They are widely used in many electronic devices, including radio and television transmitters, quart clocks, etc.

The video demonstrates the impact of sending voltage (energy) to a crystal, showing that it can vibrate and create a frequency!

Consider the profound effect when we meditate and channel our energy and intentions into a crystal. Does the crystal respond by vibrating and aligning us with that positive frequency?

Cultural Traditions

Diverse cultures have recognized and harnessed the power of gemstones for centuries:

1. **Ancient Egypt:** The Egyptians adorned themselves with lapis lazuli, carnelian, and other stones for protection, vitality, and connection to the divine.

2. **Traditional Chinese Medicine:** Jade, turquoise, and other stones were used to harmonize energies, promote healing, and balance the body's elements.

3. **Ayurveda:** The Indian tradition utilized gemstones like sapphires, rubies, and emeralds to balance the body's doshas and enhance spiritual growth.

4. **Native American Cultures:** Turquoise, quartz, and other stones were valued for their spiritual significance, healing properties, and connection to the earth.

Crystal Healing And Holistic Health

Crystal	Frequency	Potential Benefits
Amethyst	141.27 Hz	Calming, spiritual growth, intuition
Clear Quartz	327.03 Hz	Amplifying energy, clarity, healing
Rose Quartz	332.40 Hz	Love, emotional healing, self-esteem
Citrine	528 Hz	Abundance, creativity, positivity
Selenite	Varies	Cleansing, clearing energy, connecting
Lapis Lazuli	Varies	Wisdom, truth, communication
Black Tourmaline	Varies	Protection, grounding, dispelling negativity
Hematite	Varies	Grounding, focus, strength

Please note that these frequencies are based on the claims of various sources within the crystal healing community. The frequencies listed may vary depending on the source, and scientific research does not support the associations with specific benefits.

The application of gemstones for healing purposes is rooted in the belief that they can restore energetic balance, resulting in improved well-being. Though with limited scientific backing, holistic practices suggest the following benefits:

1. **Energetic Balance:** Gemstones are believed to help restore equilibrium to imbalanced energy centers (chakras) within the body.

2. **Emotional Healing:** Specific stones are associated with emotions and can assist in releasing negativity, promoting emotional growth, and enhancing self-awareness.

3. **Stress Reduction:** Gems like amethyst and rose quartz calm the mind, alleviate stress, and encourage a peaceful state of being.

4. **Physical Wellness:** Certain gemstones, like clear quartz, are thought to amplify energy and aid physical healing.

Technological and Modern Applications

Beyond holistic healing, crystals have found their way into modern technologies, showcasing their unique properties:

1. **Quartz Clocks:** Quartz's piezoelectric property is utilized in clocks and watches, providing precise timekeeping.

2. **Semiconductors:** Silicon crystals, including computer chips and solar panels, are fundamental to modern electronics.

3. **Laser Technology:** Gemstones like ruby and sapphire are used as laser mediums in medical and industrial applications.

Incorporating Gemstones for Health

Integrating gemstones into your life can be a fulfilling practice:

1. **Selection:** Choose gemstones based on your intentions and needs. Research their metaphysical properties to align with your goals.

2. **Personal Adornment:** Wear gemstone jewelry or carry small crystals to benefit from their energies throughout the day.

3. **Meditation and Visualization:** Use gemstones during meditation to amplify intentions and foster a deeper connection to your inner self. Store your gems in a sacred space, cleansing them as needed, according to their specific instructions.

4. **Crystal Grids:** Consider creating your unique geometric patterns, grids, and formations with your crystals. Arrange crystals in specific geometric patterns to enhance their combined energies and address particular concerns.

Gemstones serve as remarkable energy conduits, carrying within them a tapestry of cultural traditions, technological significance, and potential holistic benefits. By tapping into their frequencies, we can connect with the ancient wisdom of diverse cultures and explore new avenues of well-being, both within ourselves and the world around us.

Harnessing Intuition: The Power Of Developing Our Inner Sense

In a world governed by logic and reason, listening to our bodies and trusting our gut feelings might seem whimsical or impractical. Yet, recent research into **interoception**—*the inner sense that connects our minds and bodies*—reveals a complex paradox. Most importantly, it suggests that our intuition and gut feelings are not just whims but tangible skills that can be cultivated over time with focus and practice.

Take, for instance, the case of an individual who worries excessively about their heart health. Despite the temptation to dismiss their concerns as melodramatic, recent studies in neurology have shown otherwise. Sarah Garfinkel, a neuroscientist at University College London, monitored the heartbeats of individuals with autism and found that those who were initially inaccurate at sensing their heartbeats improved their accuracy over time; moreover, some participants reported that as their interoceptive ability improved, their feelings of anxiety decreased. The improvement seen in individuals with autism suggests that our inner sense of interoception is not a fixed trait but rather a skill that can be honed.

Interoception itself can be divided into three categories. The first encompasses conscious feelings driven by necessity, like knowing when to eat, sleep, or hydrate. The second includes unconscious communication between our brains and bodies, such as releasing hormones in response to changing glucose levels. The third category is about how our bodies and minds work together to sense and respond to events, highlighting the synchronicity between the two.

This third category is what we refer to when we say "listen to your body" or "trust your gut." This interoception allows us to gauge our overall mood by combining our mental state with how our organs, muscles, and nerves react to a situation. Studies have shown that individuals more attuned to their bodies outperformed others in decision-making tasks, emphasizing the value of this skill in making better decisions.

While honing our intuition sounds appealing, it's important to note that not everyone possesses the same level of interoceptive accuracy. Personal experiences, mental health conditions, and stress levels can influence our ability to accurately interpret these internal signals. The paradox lies here: although we can develop intuition, it's not a foolproof guide.

Researchers are exploring ways to train individuals' interoceptive responses to improve mental health conditions. For example, individuals with eating disorders are exposed to sensations like taste and fullness to reshape their interoceptive interpretations. New therapies like motorized capsules that vibrate when they reach the digestive system aim to enhance gastrointestinal interoception.

While cultivating intuition has its benefits, it's not a one-size-fits-all solution. Excessive focus on interoception might not always yield positive outcomes, especially for individuals with anxiety or depression. Striking a balance between tuning into our bodies and remaining open to the external world is key.

Just as artists hone their skills, we too can cultivate our inner sense to navigate life's complexities more effectively. The journey involves understanding the interplay between our minds and bodies, recognizing the potential pitfalls as they come along, and finding the right balance between introspection and engagement with the world.

Cultivating Vibrational Resonance Through Like-Minded Connections

When embarking on this journey of caring for ourselves, we must remember that we are NOT alone in our efforts. This is why it is so crucial that you do your part in seeking, attracting, aligning, and growing with like-minded individuals; moreover, the universe conspires to turn your vision into reality when you make the decision. This powerful facet of the law of attraction even applies to uniting you with people on the same vibrational waves as you!

Just as the frequencies of the universe shape our existence, we emit our unique vibrational frequencies, too. These energetic signatures, the essence of who we are, ripple outward into the world, subtly influencing the people and experiences we attract. Like a symphony seeking harmony, our vibrations align with others who resonate with our authentic selves. By embracing our true nature, we become magnets for individuals who share our passions, values, and aspirations.

In the grand cosmic dance, atoms come together, forming bonds that shape the fabric of our reality. Likewise, we witness the magnetic pull of kindred souls in our human interactions. Drawing inspiration from the scientific principle of attraction, we understand that like-minded individuals are naturally drawn to each other. When we radiate our authentic selves, we create a gravitational force that beckons those who align with our core being.

We know this force is real through our ever-expanding understanding of **neural synchronization**. The beautiful phenomenon observed when brain waves align during social interactions is a profound testament to the power of human connection. You see, as we cultivate relationships with like-minded individuals, we enter into a dance of shared understanding, empathy, and resonance. Our thoughts, emotions, and physiological responses harmonize, creating a fertile ground for growth and transformation.

When we encounter relationships exhibiting neural synchronization characteristics, we discover a profound sense of well-being and mutual support. Healthy connections foster an environment where individual growth is nurtured and collective potentials are amplified. We experience deep empathy, authentic communication, and a shared sense of purpose in these relationships. Trust, respect, and a shared journey toward self-realization become the pillars of these connections.

In this, *our vibrations echo across the universe in the symphony of life, attracting those whose souls resonate with our own.* We embark on a transformative journey of self-discovery and collective growth by seeking, attracting, aligning with, and nurturing relationships with like-minded individuals. As we witness the magic of neural synchronization unfolding within our relationships, we find solace in knowing that we are not alone on this cosmic voyage.

United in the power of resonant connections, we illuminate the world with our radiant light. I pray that, over time, we may unite to elevate the quality of light we welcome into our lives, thereby collectively upgrading our world for the better.

The Cellular Level

Our bodies are constantly undergoing cellular processes that impact our health and well-being. These processes include energy metabolism, immune system function, and DNA repair. When these processes are disrupted or inefficient, it can lead to a range of health problems.

One way to support these cellular processes and promote overall health is through healing practices that work with our biological and circadian rhythms. Our bodies have natural rhythms that govern everything from our sleep-wake cycle to our hormone production and digestion. **Circadian360** advocates healing by engaging our five senses. Through a plant-based diet protocol aligned with intermittent fasting based on the circadian rhythm, we support our body's natural processes. We can support and optimize our cellular processes by engaging in healing practices that work with these rhythms.

We must begin to accept that every sunrise gifts us a new birth, a chance to renew ourselves, align with the Earth's heartbeat, and synchronize with the universe's rhythm. When we are aligned and in harmony with our universe, we are accountable for what is within our control, actively making the best choices possible; moreover, when we start moving in sync with these rhythms, we suddenly find ourselves vibrating with others who are similarly moving while moving away from those with stagnant energy vibrations that no longer resonate with ours.

To reset and cleanse ourselves on a cellular level, it begins with acknowledging our individual mastery. *We are the architects of our own well-being.* Doctors, teachers, friends, pets, experience, plants, and environments all but mirror your growth experience as a human being. When we accept that we are the master of our internal universe, we can learn about and utilize the tools necessary for our life's growth.

Retune, Reset, And Recalibrate Your Body's Frequency By Regularly Practicing Grounding/Earthing

In an era characterized by digital distractions and urban landscapes, the ancient practice of grounding, or earthing, emerges as a powerful conduit to reconnect with Earth's profound healing energies. Scientific research, including the seminal study "Earthing: Health Implications of Reconnecting the Human Body to the Earth's Surface Electrons," illuminates the transformative potential of this practice.

Led by Clinton Ober, Dr. Stephen T. Sinatra, and Martin Zucker, this groundbreaking research explores the intricate relationship between direct contact with the Earth and human health. The study showed that grounding facilitates the transfer of electrons from the Earth's surface to the body, thus modulating inflammation and oxidative stress—a claim corroborated by findings that indicate a reduction in inflammatory markers in individuals practicing grounding.

The study indeed underscores the influence of grounding on the autonomic nervous system, illustrating its role in balancing the sympathetic and parasympathetic branches. Participants engaging in grounding exhibited enhanced heart rate variability—an indicator of improved stress response regulation and overall well-being.

The research also alludes to grounding's impact on sleep patterns and cortisol secretion. Individuals practicing grounding experienced a shift towards a balanced cortisol rhythm, contributing to improved sleep quality and overall vitality. We have discussed prior that our circadian rhythm regulates these hormones! This shows that this ancient birthright of walking outdoors is practically mandatory for biological beings on Earth to maintain basic, optimum health.

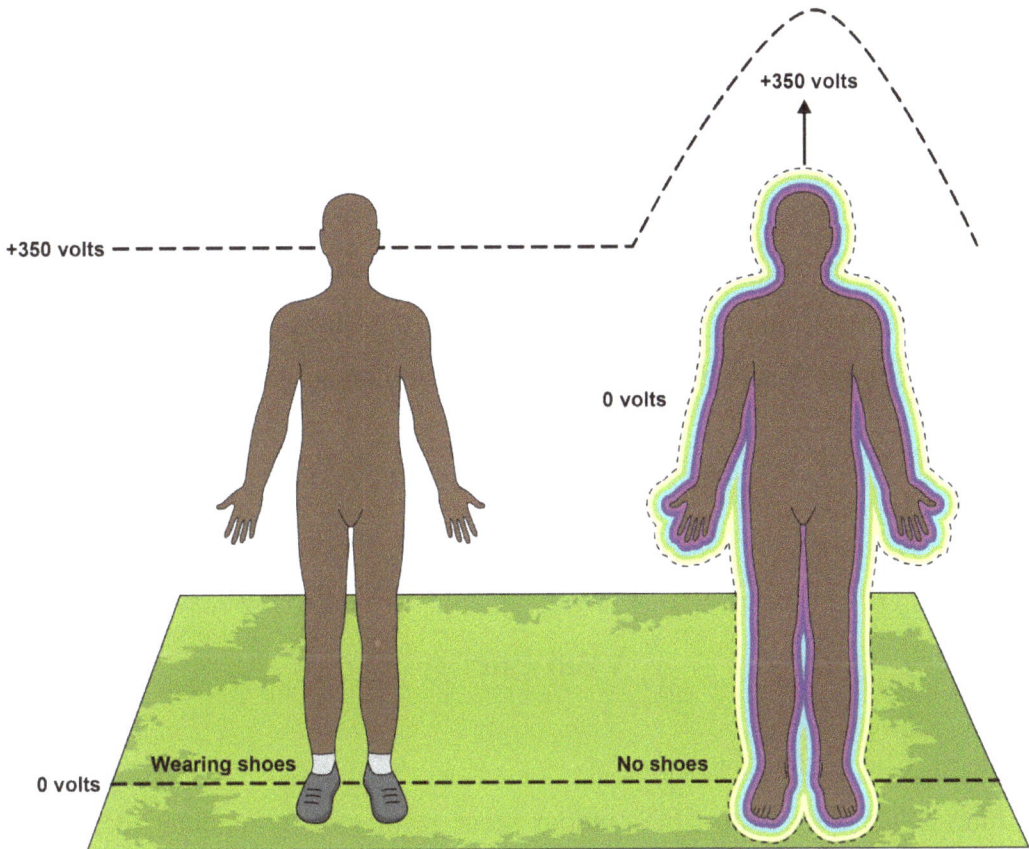

The Umbrella Effect when Earthing / Grounding

CIRCADIAN360

+350 volts

+350 volts

0 volts

Wearing shoes   No shoes

0 volts

What is exciting is that grounding's potential in mitigating the effects of electromagnetic fields finds support in the study. By aligning with Earth's natural electric field, grounding protects against ubiquitous electromagnetic radiation, potentially ameliorating its impact on our health. Seriously, also known as **"the umbrella effect,"** when a person is barefoot on the ground, particularly if the ground is moist, such as grass or soil, their body can become electrically conductive. Electrons from the Earth can flow into the person's body, equalizing the electrical potential. Wearing shoes, especially rubber or synthetic soles, can act as insulators, preventing the easy flow of electrons between the Earth and the person's body. As a result, the person's body might not experience the same level of electrical connection with the Earth's surface as when barefoot.

The implications of this research extend beyond the theoretical, aligning with centuries-old practices observed by indigenous cultures. As we traverse an era of unprecedented technological advancement, the wisdom of grounding beckons us to reconnect with the Earth's energies—a practice that science now backs as a gateway to enhanced well-being.

Incorporating grounding into our daily lives invites us to unlock vitality, boost resilience, and foster a more profound harmony between human biology and the natural world. As we stand on the precipice of this knowledge, the insights from "Earthing: Health Implications of Reconnecting the Human Body to the Earth's Surface Electrons" illuminate a path toward a more vibrant, balanced, and connected existence.

A Guide To Grounding Your Body: Reconnecting With Earth's Vital Energy

Step 1: Choose the Right Spot

Find a safe and comfortable outdoor space to practice grounding. Ideal places include grassy lawns, sandy beaches, and unpaved pathways. Ensure the area is free from debris, sharp objects, and potential hazards.

Step 2: Dress Comfortably

Wear comfortable clothing that allows direct skin contact with the Earth (consider wearing high frequency garments as described earlier in this book0. Avoid insulating materials like rubber or synthetic fabrics, as these can prevent the transfer of electrons from the Earth to your body.

Step 3: Breathe and Center Yourself

Stand or sit comfortably in your chosen spot. Take a few deep, slow breaths to relax your body and mind. Allow any stress or tension to melt away as you prepare to connect with the Earth's energy.

Step 4: Go Barefoot or Use Natural Materials

If possible, take off your shoes and socks. Feel the Earth beneath your feet, allowing the direct contact to initiate the energy flow. If you cannot go barefoot, use natural materials like cotton or leather footwear that allow electrons to pass through.

Step 5: Absorb Earth's Energy

Stand, sit, or lie on the ground, maintaining direct contact with the Earth's surface. Imagine roots extending from your body into the Earth, anchoring you securely. Feel the sensations of the ground beneath you, whether it's the coolness of grass, the warmth of the sand, or the texture of the soil.

Step 6: Engage Your Senses

Engage your senses to deepen your connection with nature. Feel the Earth's textures, listen to the sounds around you, and observe the beauty of your surroundings. Let go of distractions and immerse yourself in the present moment.

Step 7: Stay Present

Spend at least 15-30 minutes grounding yourself, although longer sessions can be even more beneficial. Use this time to meditate, practice deep breathing, or enjoy the stillness of nature. In the Circadian360 Mindfulness & Manifestations Workbook, the Daily Sunrise Illuminations Ritual Checklist invites you to use this time while grounding, to actively complete provided worksheets designed to help support your overall mental health and well-being.

Step 8: Gently Release

When you're ready to conclude your grounding practice, do so gently. Slowly stand up or sit up, taking a moment to acknowledge the energy exchange that has taken place. Express gratitude for this opportunity to connect with the Earth.

Step 9: Integrate Grounding into Your Routine

Incorporate grounding into your daily routine whenever possible. Take breaks during work to step outside and connect with nature. Engage in barefoot walks, picnics, or outdoor activities that allow you to stay rooted in the Earth's energy.

Step 10: Observe the Effects

Pay attention to how grounding affects your well-being over time. Many people report improved sleep, reduced stress, increased energy, reduction in pain resulting from nerve damage, and a heightened sense of calm after engaging in regular grounding practices. If you notice sciatic pain, lower back pain, foot discomfort and stiffness in the body arising due to too much sitting, poor hydration and/or lack of exercise, please make sure that you treat yourself to a walk in the park, have a picnic on some green grass and lay down on your favorite blanket outside!

By following these steps and embracing the practice of grounding, you can tap into the Earth's abundant energy, release accumulated stress, and restore your body's natural equilibrium. Allow the Earth to support you in your journey toward holistic well-being, and revel in the connection between humans and nature since the dawn of time.

The Circadian Rhythm Clock

CIRCADIAN360'S BODY CLOCK

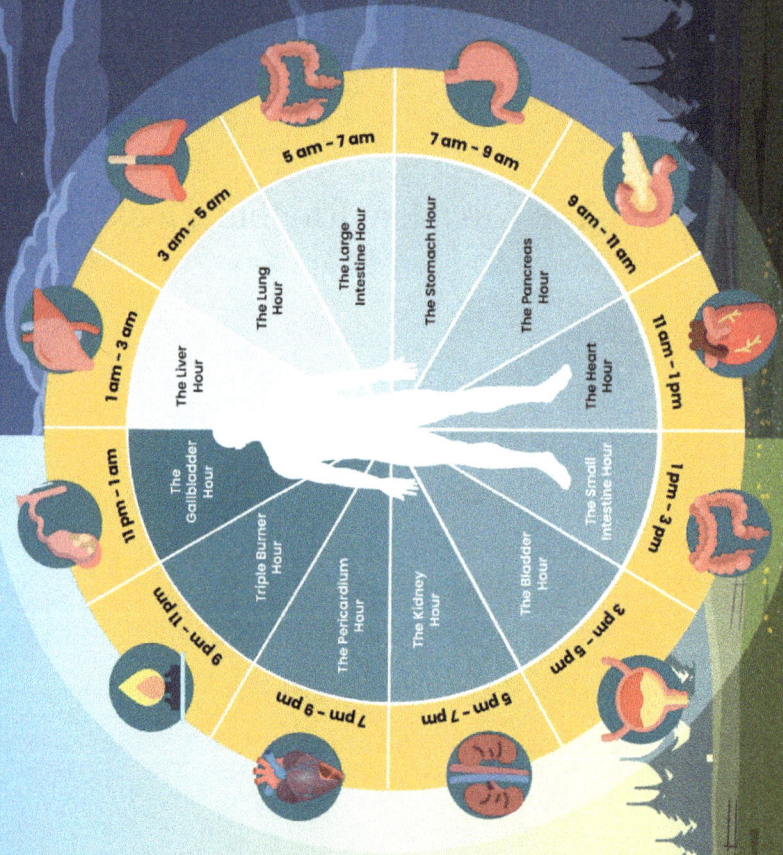

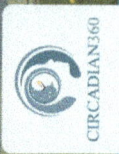

The Liver Hour — 1 am – 3 am
The Lung Hour — 3 am – 5 am
The Large Intestine Hour — 5 am – 7 am
The Stomach Hour — 7 am – 9 am
The Pancreas Hour — 9 am – 11 am
The Heart Hour — 11 am – 1pm
The Small Intestine Hour — 1 pm – 3 pm
The Bladder Hour — 3 pm – 5 pm
The Kidney Hour — 5 pm – 7 pm
The Pericardium Hour — 7 pm – 9 pm
Triple Burner Hour — 9 pm – 11 pm
The Gallbladder Hour — 11 pm – 1 am

CIRCADIAN360

CIRCADIAN360'S BODY CLOCK

1 am - 3 am: THE LIVER HOUR
Body Functions: Liver detoxification, blood regeneration, and hormone regulation
Body Meridian Point: Liver (LR1)
Things to Do: Get plenty of rest, avoid heavy meals and alcohol, practice relaxation techniques
Things to Avoid: Strenuous activities, intense emotions, working late into the night

5 am - 7 am: THE LARGE INTESTINE HOUR
Body Functions: Large intestine detoxification, elimination, and hydration
Body Meridian Point: Large Intestine (LI1)
Things to Do: Drink plenty of water, practice gentle stretching exercises, avoid late-night snacks
Things to Avoid: Excessive consumption of alcohol, spicy or fatty foods, negative thoughts

9 am - 11 am: THE PANCREAS HOUR
Body Functions: Pancreatic detoxification, hormone regulation, and blood sugar control
Body Meridian Point: Spleen (SP3)
Things to Do: Eat a healthy breakfast, practice moderate exercises, take a walk in the sun
Things to Avoid: Skipping breakfast, eating sugary or processed foods, rushing or overworking

3 am - 5 am: THE LUNG HOUR
Body Functions: Lung detoxification, oxygenation, and immune function
Body Meridian Point: Lung (LU8)
Things to Do: Get plenty of rest, practice deep breathing exercises, avoid exposure to pollutants
Things to Avoid: Smoking, consumption of dairy products, working late into the night

7 am - 9 am: THE STOMACH HOUR
Body Functions: Stomach detoxification, nutrient absorption, and energy production
Body Meridian Point: Stomach (ST36)
Things to Do: Eat a healthy breakfast, practice gentle exercises, avoid skipping meals
Things to Avoid: Eating heavy or greasy foods, drinking too much caffeine, excessive mental stress

11 am - 1 pm: THE HEART HOUR
Body Functions: Heart detoxification, blood circulation, and emotional regulation
Body Meridian Point: Heart (HT8)
Things to Do: Take a break, practice relaxation techniques, express gratitude and joy
Things to Avoid: Overworking, excessive mental stress, consuming caffeinated beverages

1 pm - 3 pm: THE SMALL INTESTINE HOUR
Body Functions: Small intestine detoxification, nutrient absorption, and digestion
Body Meridian Point: Small Intestine (SI5)
Things to Do: Eat a healthy lunch, practice moderate exercises, take a break from work
Things to Avoid: Eating too quickly, consuming heavy or greasy foods, skipping meals

5 pm - 7 pm: THE KIDNEY HOUR
Body Meridian Point: Kidney (KI10)
Things to Do: Drink plenty of water, practice gentle exercises, take a short break to rest your eyes
Things to Avoid: Excessive consumption of caffeine or alcohol, working too intensely, holding onto neg

9 pm - 11 pm: THE TRIPLE BURNER HOUR
Body Functions: Triple Burner detoxification, hormone regulation, and metabolism
Body Meridian Point: Triple Burner / San Jiao (SJ6)
Things to Do: Have a light dinner, wind down with calming activities, spend quality time with loved ones
Things to Avoid: Eating heavy or greasy foods, watching TV or using electronic devices before bed, overthinking

3 pm - 5 pm: THE BLADDER HOUR
Body Functions: Bladder detoxification, fluid regulation, and hormone production
Body Meridian Point: Bladder (BL66)
Things to Do: Drink plenty of water, take a short nap or rest, practice relaxation techniques
Things to Avoid: Drinking too much caffeine, holding urine for too long, overexertion

7 pm - 9 pm: THE PERICARDIUM HOUR
Body Functions: Pericardium detoxification, emotional regulation, and circulation
Body Meridian Point: Pericardium (PC6)
Things to Do: Practice self-care, spend time with loved ones, do something enjoyable
Things to Avoid: Overworking, excessive stress, skipping meals or snacks

11 pm - 1 am: THE GALLBLADDER HOUR
Body Functions: Gallbladder detoxification, digestion, and hormone regulation
Body Meridian Point: Gallbladder (GB41)
Things to Do: Prepare for bed, practice relaxation techniques, avoid late-night snacking
Things to Avoid: Eating heavy or greasy foods, consuming caffeine or alcohol, working late into the night

CIRCADIAN360

The Nobel Prize was awarded in 2017 to Jeffrey C. Hall, Michael Rosbash, and Michael W. Young for their breakthrough discovery that shed light on the genetic basis of circadian rhythms. These rhythms refer to the physical, mental, and behavioral changes that occur over a 24-hour cycle and are influenced by light and darkness. Studying these rhythms is known as chronobiology; they affect almost all living organisms, including animals, plants, and microbes.

Crucial genes establishing the body's natural clock are the Period and Cryptochrome genes, which produce proteins that accumulate in the cell's nucleus at night and decrease during the day. Studies on fruit flies have shown that these proteins play a vital role in regulating feelings of wakefulness, alertness, and sleepiness; however, external factors such as exposure to light at different times of day can also impact circadian rhythms.

Sunlight serves as a vital cue for the brain's internal clock, known as the suprachiasmatic nucleus (SCN), and the clock then determines when these various functions occur in the body. Beyond sleep-wake cycles, circadian rhythms significantly influence metabolism, heart rate, blood pressure, and much more. They even play a role in regulating blood sugar, cholesterol, mental health conditions, immune system function, DNA repair, and even the effectiveness of cancer treatments.

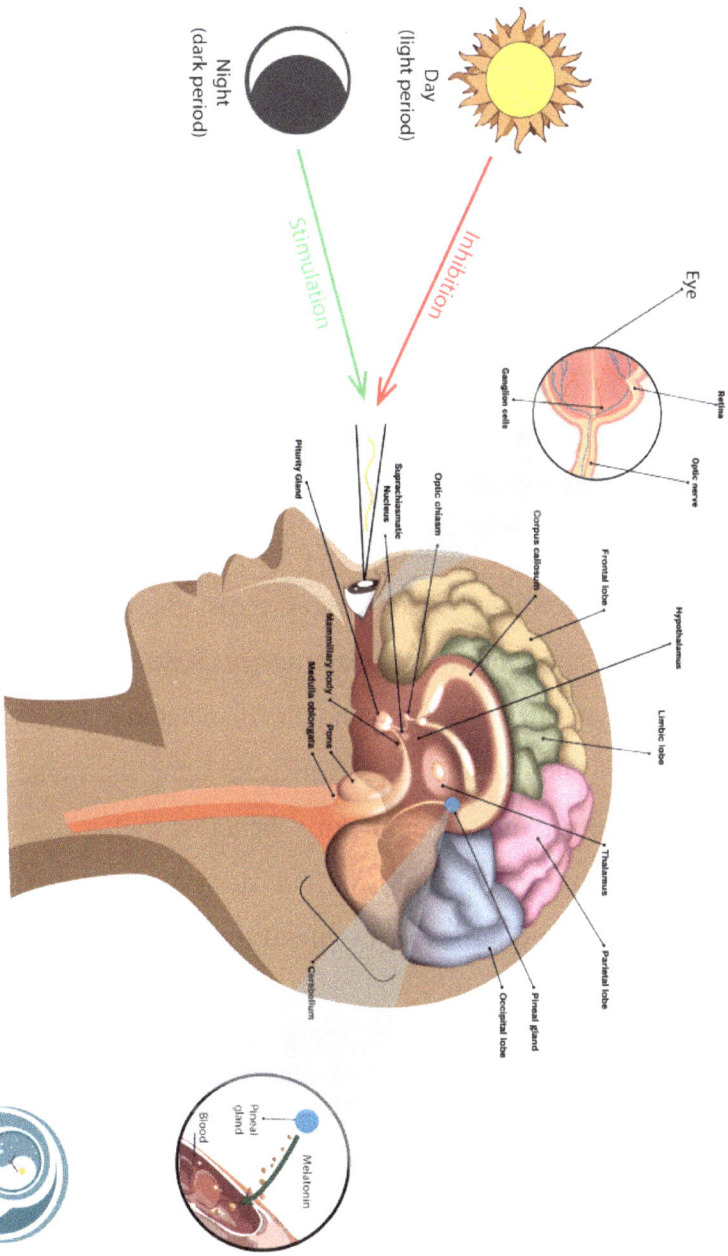

Circadian360's The CIRCADIAN MIND

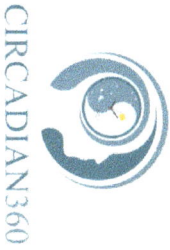

Day (light period)

Night (dark period)

Inhibition

Stimulation

Eye

Ganglion cells

Retina

Optic nerve

Pituitary Gland

Suprachiasmatic Nucleus

Optic chiasm

Corpus callosum

Frontal lobe

Hypothalamus

Limbic lobe

Mammillary body

Medulla oblongata

Pons

Thalamus

Parietal lobe

Cerebellum

Pineal gland

Occipital lobe

Pineal gland

Blood

Melatonin

CIRCADIAN360

Just as professional athletes tend to lose their expert abilities over time, our circadian rhythm becomes less efficient the older we get; moreover, due to the overconsumption of electronic devices emitting blue light and late-night eating, we are finding a phenomenon where younger people live with less efficient circadian rhythms. This is known as "the flattening" of the circadian rhythm. It was proven in 2017 through research conducted by Susan Hood and Shimon Amir in their paper "The Again Clock: Circadian Rhythms and Later Life - PMID:28145903".

As we age, the body's circadian rhythm undergoes many changes, including dampening the circadian hormones melatonin and cortisol, reduced circadian signaling through the eyes and brain, and shorter and more fragmented sleep cycles. Research also finds that individuals over the age of 65 tend to sleep significantly less than those in their younger years. This is primarily due to the results of circadian system damage, as found in the 2004 research by Maurice M Ohayon et al. "Meta-analysis of quantitative sleep parameters from childhood to old age in health individuals: developing normative sleep values across the human lifespan - PMID: 15586779". This happens because our melatonin levels decrease with age, and older individuals produce a significantly less amount of melatonin than younger people. When we honor that melatonin is also an anti-aging hormone, the strongest antioxidant, has powerful anti-inflammatory benefits, helps regulate longevity, promotes cellular repair, and has cardio and neuroprotective benefits, we can understand that lower melatonin levels eventually will result in less cellular repair and faster aging.

While many may think melatonin is related to sleep, it also supports apoptosis, autophagy, brain detoxing, bone health, immune health, fat burning, and cognitive wellness/memory health.

The pineal gland in the brain produces the often under-appreciated melatonin hormone. It's often referred to as the "sleep hormone" because its levels typically rise in the evening, signaling to the body that it's time to prepare for sleep. Exposure to natural light, especially in the morning, suppresses melatonin production. This is part of the body's way of promoting wakefulness during the day. In the evening, melatonin production increases as the sunlight becomes dimmer and has less of it's blue component. This rise in melatonin levels helps promote sleepiness and prepares the body for restorative sleep.

Usually, disruptions to biological rhythms occur due to natural changes in age or environmental factors; however, it seems that since the 3rd Industrial Revolution, more unnatural disruptions have emerged in our world, helping to both give rise to and feed epidemics in cardiovascular disease, metabolic health, cancer, depression, anxiety, insomnia, neurological disorders, immune function, and both genetic and epigenetic concerns. For instance, with the advent of airplanes has come jet lag disorder caused by travel across time zones; moreover, with more demands on the labor economy, we now have an epidemic in shift work disorder stemming from non-traditional work schedules (working 8-12+ hours shifts and/or overnight hours).

A more alarming phenomenon comes from artificial blue light exposure. The blue light you see in the sky due to Rayleigh scattering is related to the blue light emitted by LED (Light Emitting Diode) lights. Both types of blue light have a similar appearance because they involve light in the blue part of the visible spectrum. The blue light in the sky is natural sunlight scattered by the Earth's atmosphere, while LED lights are artificial sources containing blue light created using semiconductor technology. LED lights can be much more intense and concentrated compared to the relatively diffuse blue light from the sky. This intensity can have significant adverse effects on our overall health.

Blue light emitted from screens tricks the brain into perceiving it as daylight, thus suppressing melatonin production and making it challenging to fall asleep. Even with older tube-style televisions, staring at the TV screen for extended periods, especially late at night, contributed to sleep disruptions; moreover, contingent on the television program, computer application, website, app, social media platform, texting service, and/or even your LED nightlights and household lightbulbs, the continual excitation and stimulation keeps the brain engaged and alert.

Understanding our circadian rhythm can help optimize your daily routines and support your overall health and wellness. By recognizing the peak times of day for specific organ systems, individuals can tailor their daily activities (exercising, eating, sleeping, etc) to align with their body's natural rhythms. Following these guidelines can improve physical, emotional, and mental health, leading to a more balanced and harmonious life.

You will notice that the body's meridian system is acknowledged in **Circadian360's Body Clock**. In Traditional Chinese Medicine (TCM), Meridians are channels or pathways through which vital energy, known as Qi (pronounced Chee), flows throughout the body. These meridians form a complex network connecting various organs, systems, and tissues. Depending on the source, there are typically 12 main meridians displayed in TCM, each associated with specific organs and functions. The flow of Qi along these meridians is believed to regulate and maintain the overall balance and health of the body. For more detailed information on meridians, including their specific pathways and connections, please refer to the *Healing Using the Five Sense: Self-Care Routines & Hacks* sections of this book, where you can explore the concept of meridians in a directly applicable way.

Here is an outline of the different hours, corresponding body functions, Chinese medicine meridians, and things to do and avoid during particular daily intervals:

1 am - 3 am: The Liver Hour

Body Functions: Liver detoxification, blood regeneration, and hormone regulation.

Body Meridian Point: Liver (LR1)

Things to Do: Get plenty of rest, avoid heavy meals and alcohol, and practice relaxation techniques.

Things to Avoid: Strenuous activities, intense emotions, working late into the night.

3 am - 5 am: The Lung Hour

Body Functions: Lung detoxification, oxygenation, and immune function.

Body Meridian Point: Lung (LU8)

Things to Do: Get plenty of rest, practice deep breathing exercises, and avoid pollutant exposure.

Things to Avoid: Smoking, consumption of dairy products, working late into the night.

5 am - 7 am: The Large Intestine Hour

Body Functions: Large intestine detoxification, elimination, and hydration.

Body Meridian Point: Large Intestine (LI1)

Things to Do: Drink plenty of water, practice gentle stretching exercises, avoid late-night snacks

Things to Avoid: Excessive consumption of alcohol, spicy or fatty foods, negative thoughts

7 am - 9 am: The Stomach Hour

Body Functions: Stomach detoxification, nutrient absorption, and energy production

Body Meridian Point: Stomach (ST36)

Things to Do: Eat a healthy breakfast, practice gentle exercises, avoid skipping meals

Things to Avoid: Eating heavy or greasy foods, drinking too much caffeine, excessive mental stress

9 am - 11 am: The Pancreas Hour

Body Functions: Pancreatic detoxification, hormone regulation, and blood sugar control

Body Meridian Point: Spleen (SP3)

Things to Do: Eat a healthy breakfast, practice moderate exercises, take a walk in the sun

Things to Avoid: Skipping breakfast, eating sugary or processed foods, rushing or overworking

11 am - 1 pm: The Heart Hour

Body Functions: Heart detoxification, blood circulation, and emotional regulation

Body Meridian Point: Heart (HT8)

Things to Do: Take a break, practice relaxation techniques, express gratitude and joy

Things to Avoid: Overworking, excessive mental stress, consuming caffeinated beverages

1 pm - 3 pm: The Small Intestine Hour

Body Functions: Small intestine detoxification, nutrient absorption, and digestion

Body Meridian Point: Small Intestine (SI5)

Things to Do: Eat a healthy lunch, practice moderate exercises, take a break from work

Things to Avoid: Eating too quickly, consuming heavy or greasy foods, skipping meals

3 pm - 5 pm: The Bladder Hour

Body Functions: Bladder detoxification, fluid regulation, and hormone production

Body Meridian Point: Bladder (BL66)

Things to Do: Drink plenty of water, take a short nap or rest, practice relaxation techniques

Things to Avoid: Drinking too much caffeine, holding urine for too long, overexertion

5 pm - 7 pm: The Kidney Hour

Body Meridian Point: Kidney (KI10)

Things to Do: Drink plenty of water, practice gentle exercises, and take a short break to rest your eyes

Things to Avoid: Excessive consumption of caffeine or alcohol, working too intensely, holding onto negative emotions

7 pm - 9 pm: The Pericardium Hour

Body Functions: Pericardium detoxification, emotional regulation, and circulation

Body Meridian Point: Pericardium (PC8)

Things to Do: Practice self-care, spend time with loved ones, do something enjoyable

Things to Avoid: Overworking, excessive stress, skipping meals or snacks

9 pm - 11 pm: The Triple Burner Hour

Body Functions: Triple Burner detoxification, hormone regulation, and metabolism

Body Meridian Point: Triple Burner / San Jiao (SJ6)

Things to Do: Have a light dinner, wind down with calming activities, spend quality time with loved ones

Things to Avoid: Eating heavy or greasy foods, watching TV or using electronic devices before bed, overthinking

11 pm - 1 am: The Gallbladder Hour

Body Functions: Gallbladder detoxification, digestion, and hormone regulation

Body Meridian Point: Gallbladder (GB41)

Things to Do: Prepare for bed, practice relaxation techniques, avoid late-night snacking

Things to Avoid: Eating heavy or greasy foods, consuming caffeine or alcohol, working late into the night

A combination of genetic history, unique experiences, and our choices shapes each of us. These factors profoundly impact our quality of life. In **Circadian360**, we embrace the notion that we are fully responsible for our healing journey. We understand that true healing goes beyond merely treating symptoms with medications or herbs, recognizing that healing entails delving into the root causes of our health challenges and making the essential adjustments. We embark on a transformative path toward holistic healing and personal growth by conducting thorough self-health assessments and cultivating genuine self-acceptance of our well-being.

Learned Helplessness, Neglect, and Self-Neglect Are The First Root Causes Of Illness

Through the writings of pioneering herbalist Hannah Kroeger, I was first introduced to the truth that neglect can be a root cause of illness, disease, and ill health. Individuals must take responsibility for their health by understanding their body's basic functions and needs, treating it as the sacred temple it truly is; however, it is often through a lack of knowledge, resources, education, or even apathy that individuals develop and maintain unhealthy habits that contribute to self-neglect.

An exciting example of this can be seen in a classic experiment by G.C. Williams in the 1957 study conducted on fleas. The study revealed that fleas, when placed in a jar with a lid on it, would continue to jump but eventually stop attempting to leave captivity. This phenomenon is known as "learned helplessness," where an organism accepts the limitations of its environment and stops trying to escape or change its circumstances. Even once the lid was removed, the fleas would only continue to jump just to the point of where the lid once was, never leaving the jar. Similarly, individuals may not even realize the limitations of their environments or the impact of their habits on their health, leading to **self-neglect**.

Self-neglect manifests as behaviors or habits where individuals disregard their physical and mental health needs. In other words, when someone is not taking care of themselves, they engage in self-neglect. This can lead to various health issues and diseases if not appropriately addressed. We must understand our body's basic needs, such as proper nutrition, exercise, and rest, and treat our body like the ultimate temple. If we don't, we are putting ourselves at risk of self-neglect and ultimately hurting our health.

Continuously seeking knowledge and education is our shield against self-neglect, and with each new piece of understanding, we leap higher, reaching for better health and well-being. We aren't bound by the lifestyle choices of our parents, and ignorance in the past should not shackle our future. Embracing knowledge empowers us to break free from harmful patterns, fostering a healthier, more vibrant life; moreover, the individuals and families who adapt their unhealthy traditions into healthy and enduring ones will ultimately survive the longest.

Getting To Know Your Body AND The Body's Basic Functioning Needs

As we open the lid to this jar of wellness, we first must start with the basics- the building blocks of human life.

Minerals

These inorganic substances, present in the earth and water around us, are the proper foundation of our physical makeup. They serve as the bricks and mortar of every cell within our bodies, forming the structural framework upon which all other biological processes depend. Without minerals, our bodies could not perform even the most basic functions necessary for survival. So, while we may take the importance of vitamins and other nutrients for granted, our humble mineral-friends truly deserve our appreciation and attention.

They play essential roles in everything from bone health and muscle function to nerve and hormone regulation. Some examples of essential minerals include calcium, iron, and magnesium.

The human body needs at least 16 essential minerals to function properly. These include:

- Calcium
- Chloride
- Chromium

- Copper
- Fluoride
- Iodine
- Iron
- Magnesium
- Manganese
- Molybdenum
- Phosphorus
- Potassium
- Selenium
- Sodium
- Sulfur
- Zinc

These minerals are necessary for various bodily functions, such as building strong bones, maintaining a healthy immune system, regulating blood pressure, and producing energy. A balanced diet that includes a variety of whole foods can help ensure the body gets the minerals it needs.

Here's the list of minerals with their descriptions in alphabetical order:

1. BORON: Inadequate boron intake has been associated with poor absorption of calcium, magnesium, and phosphorus, as well as osteoporosis. Food sources of boron include fruits such as apples, pears, grapes, nuts, and legumes. Some herbs and spices, such as turmeric and ginger, contain boron.

2. CALCIUM: Insufficient calcium intake can lead to a range of symptoms such as aching joints, brittle nails, elevated blood cholesterol, heart palpitations, hypertension, insomnia, muscle cramps, nervousness, rheumatoid arthritis, rickets, tooth decay, depression, delusions, hyperactivity, and eczema. Good food sources of calcium include dairy products, leafy green vegetables, fish, and nuts. Herbs such as dandelion and nettle are also high in calcium.

3. CARBON: Carbon deficiency has been linked to a range of symptoms such as vitiligo, memory loss, anxiety, low energy, vitamin D deficiency, tiredness, anemia, loss of bone density, bone pain, muscle weakness, depression, and hair loss. Carbon is naturally obtained from food sources such as fruits, vegetables, grains, and meats. Some mushrooms, such as shiitake and maitake/hen of the woods, are also carbon-rich.

4. CHLORIDE: Chloride works alongside sodium to maintain fluid balance and electrolyte levels in the body. It is often found in table salt and many processed foods. This mineral also aids in digestion by participating in the production of stomach acid. It's commonly found in foods like olives, lettuce, and tomatoes. Some herbs like basil and thyme also provide chloride.

5. CHROMIUM: Low chromium levels have been associated with anxiety, fatigue, glucose intolerance, inadequate metabolism of minerals related to bone and muscle growth, and increased risk of arteriosclerosis. Chromium-rich foods include broccoli, potatoes, whole grains, and spices such as cinnamon and black pepper.

6. COPPER: Copper deficiency can lead to osteoporosis, anemia, baldness, diarrhea, general weakness, brain dysfunction, impaired respiratory function, and skin sores. Good food sources of copper include pomegranates, organ meats, shellfish, nuts, seeds, and leafy green vegetables. Some herbs, such as parsley and thyme, are also high in copper.

7. FLUORIDE: Fluoride is crucial for maintaining strong teeth and preventing dental cavities. It promotes enamel remineralization and helps make teeth more resistant to decay. Fluoride is often found in fluoridated water, toothpaste, and certain foods. Balanced fluoride consumption supports oral health, but excessive intake can lead to dental fluorosis. Certain herbs, like peppermint and chamomile, also contain fluoride.

8. GERANIUM: Low levels of geranium have been linked to poor cellular oxygenation and a weakened immune system, making cells more vulnerable to toxins and poisons. Good food sources of geranium include citrus fruits, apples, grapes, and nuts. Some herbs, such as rose and lemon balm, also contain geranium.

9. IODINE: Inadequate iodine intake has been linked to hormonal imbalances, breast cancer, endocrine disruption, fatigue, under-active thyroid, hypothyroidism, and weight gain. Good food sources of iodine include seaweed, fish, dairy products, and eggs. Some herbs, such as bladderwrack and nettle, also contain iodine.

10. IRON: Iron deficiency can lead to anemia, brittle hair, difficulty swallowing, digestive disturbances, dizziness, fatigue, fragile bones, hair loss, inflammation of tissues in the mouth, spoon-shaped or ridged nails, nervousness, obesity, pallor, and slowed mental reactions. Good food sources of iron include red meat, poultry, fish, leafy green vegetables, and beans. Herbs such as nettle and yellow dock are also high in iron.

11. MAGNESIUM: Low magnesium levels have been linked to confusion, muscular dystrophy, insomnia, irritability, poor digestion, rapid heartbeat, and seizures. Magnesium deficiency is associated with cardiovascular problems, asthma, depression, insomnia, chronic fatigue, and irritable bowel syndrome. Good food sources of magnesium include leafy green vegetables, nuts, seeds, fish, and whole grains. Herbs such as chamomile and passionflower are also high in magnesium.

12. MANGANESE: Low levels of manganese can result in various health problems such as memory loss, tremors, and confusion. Consuming foods rich in manganese, such as pineapple, spinach, sweet potato, and pumpkin seeds, can help prevent deficiency. Herbs like cinnamon, cloves, and turmeric are also good sources of manganese.

13. MOLYBDENUM: Molybdenum deficiency is rare but can cause mouth and gum disorders and increase the risk of brain cancer. Foods high in molybdenum include beans, lentils, peanuts, and whole grains. Shiitake mushrooms and spinach are also excellent sources of this mineral.

14. POTASSIUM: Low potassium levels may cause chills, constipation, and cognitive impairment. Consuming foods like bananas, avocados, sweet potatoes, and leafy greens can help boost potassium levels. Herbs such as basil and sage, as well as mushrooms like crimini and oyster, are also good sources of potassium.

15. PHOSPHORUS: Inadequate phosphorus intake can lead to fatigue, numbness, and irregular breathing. Foods such as salmon, beef, chicken, and dairy products are high in phosphorus. You can also get this mineral from herbs like parsley and dill and mushrooms such as portobello and shiitake.

16. SELENIUM: Deficiency of selenium has been linked to various health issues such as heart disease, fatigue, and a weakened immune system. You can get selenium from foods like Brazil nuts, tuna, and mushrooms such as shiitake and button mushrooms. Herbs such as thyme and chives also contain this mineral.

17. SILICA: Silica is vital for bone and connective tissue formation and maintaining healthy nails, skin, and hair. It can be found in oats, bananas, and green beans. Horsetail herb is an excellent source of silica and can be consumed as a tea. You can also get silica from mushrooms such as shiitake and portobello.

18. SODIUM: Adequate sodium intake is crucial for maintaining proper fluid balance, nerve transmission, and muscle function. It also plays a role in regulating blood pressure. Common sources of sodium include table salt, processed foods, and certain condiments. Balanced consumption is essential, as excessive sodium intake can lead to high blood pressure and other health issues.

The standard table salt is dangerous, and the human body needs premium, natural sea salt (as found in nature), as it contains the magnesium and all other minerals the body requires from water. The best sea salts recommended:

Celtic Salt - Celtic salt is a treasure trove of minerals and boasts a unique pH balance that distinguishes it within the world of salts. Its distinctive composition includes many trace minerals and electrolytes, resulting in various flavors and benefits. With its intriguing **pH balance of 8.14**, its mineral-rich profile boasts a captivating array of essential elements, trace minerals, and electrolytes, forming a harmonious symphony within the salt. With a **sodium chloride content of 88%**, Celtic salt separates itself from conventional table salts that often comprise a higher percentage of sodium chloride.

Himalayan Salt - Renowned for its remarkable characteristics, Himalayan salt emerges as a genuinely exceptional mineral-rich option. Himalayan salt presents a unique mineral composition exhibiting distinctive attributes, including a treasure trove of essential trace minerals and electrolytes and a **pH balance of 7.0 to 7.5**. With approximately **98% sodium chloride and an intriguing 2% comprising an array of naturally occurring trace minerals**, this salt possesses an intriguing contrast to conventional table salts. The allure of Himalayan salt lies in its mineral content and captivating pale pink hue, a testament to its origin and the ancient sea beds from which it's sourced.

Hawaiian Alaea Salt – It is an exquisite coarse salt celebrated for its distinct qualities, including a naturally lower sodium content, elevated levels of trace minerals and electrolytes, and a remarkable **pH balance of 9.37**. This salt boasts a sodium chloride content of 81%, accompanied by an impressive 19% comprised **of 80 naturally present trace minerals**. These attributes set it apart from conventional table salts, which often contain up to 99% sodium chloride. Red Alaea is also rich in iron oxides, which makes for a great digestible form of dietary iron and a minor source of copper. The coarse Alaea Red Sea Salt is a tribute to Hawaii's extraordinary landscapes, embodying the essence of baked red Alaea clay derived from within the intricate layers of lava rocks. Traditionally, Hawaiians use Alaea in healing rituals and ceremonies to cleanse, purify, and bless tools and canoes.

<u>Based on pH, sodium chloride content, percentage, and amount of naturally present trace minerals, Hawaiian Alaea Salt is a perfect sea salt from the USA.</u>

19. SULFUR: Sulfur is essential for synthesizing collagen, which helps maintain skin integrity. Foods like garlic, onions, and eggs are good sources of sulfur. Consuming mushrooms such as shiitake and portobello can also help increase sulfur intake. Natural thermal spring water is also abundant in sulfur.

20. ZINC: Zinc is essential for immune system function, wound healing, and proper growth and development. It also supports various enzymatic reactions in the body. Zinc-rich foods include meat, poultry, dairy products, nuts, and legumes. Ensuring adequate zinc intake is essential for overall health. Herbs such as oregano and sage also contain zinc.

Here is an easy cheat sheet for remembering these:
- Blood = Iron
- Liver = Copper
- Thyroid = Iodine
- Heart = Magnesium
- Pancreas = Chromium
- Adrenals & Prostate = Zinc
- Bones & Connective Tissues = Calcium

Powerhouse Sources Of Minerals:

Superfoods:

1. **Spirulina:** A blue-green Algae rich in protein, vitamins, and minerals such as iron, calcium, magnesium, and potassium.

2. **Chlorella:** Another green Alga packed with vitamins, minerals, and antioxidants, including iron, zinc, and magnesium.

3. **Kelp:** A type of seaweed that's a great source of iodine and other minerals like calcium, magnesium, and potassium.

4. **Bee Pollen:** Contains a wide range of nutrients, including minerals like calcium, magnesium, potassium, iron, and zinc.

5. **Cacao:** Raw cacao contains minerals like magnesium, iron, zinc, copper, and antioxidants.

Algae:

1. **Dulse**: A red Algae rich in minerals such as iodine, iron, magnesium, and potassium.

2. **Nori:** Another type of red Algae commonly used in sushi, providing minerals like iodine, calcium, and iron.

3. **Chondrus Crispus (Sea Moss):** Contains iodine, iron, calcium, potassium, and sulfur, among other nutrients.

Mushrooms:

1. **Reishi:** Known as the "mushroom of longevity & immortality," it offers various minerals, including potassium, calcium, and magnesium.

2. **Lion's Mane:** Rich in potassium, zinc, and other minerals, as well as compounds that may support brain health.

3. **Cordyceps:** This mushroom is known for its potential to support energy and stamina. It contains minerals like zinc, iron, and magnesium.

4. **Turkey Tail:** Known for its immune-boosting properties, turkey tail mushroom contains various minerals like potassium and selenium.

Cell Salts

Cell salts are homeopathic remedies made of certain mineral compounds found in all living things. A German doctor and homeopath, Dr. William Schuessler, developed these salts over a century ago. He discovered 12 mineral compounds vital to proper cell functioning, calling them cell salts or tissue salts. Deficiencies of these 12 mineral salts can lead to diseases and abnormal states in the body. Supplying the body with the correct combination of minerals can restore wholeness and balance, and the body can heal itself.

Tissue salts are a natural healing modality that is versatile and available over the counter at health food stores. They are inexpensive, long-lasting, and safe for home prescribing. Cell salts reinforce their corresponding field, unlike homeopathic remedies, which repel a vibrational illness in the body. Made in a 6x potency, they strengthen and nourish at a cellular level.

Cell salts enable cells to assimilate better and utilize the mineral compounds they represent in homeopathic potency. They can be used to replace a lost or needed mineral and assimilate nutrients from diet or supplementation. For example, in the case of a broken bone, taking the tissue salt caliphs can help supply a safe source of calcium and help the body assimilate and use the calcium taken in through foods high in calcium.

The dosage of cell salts is different depending on the condition. For acute conditions such as colds or cases of flu, dosing often and spreading it further until no symptoms remain is recommended. For chronic conditions such as arthritis or diabetes, taking the cell salt 2-3 times a day for three months or more is recommended.

Later, the concept of cell salts was associated with astrology by George Carey, an American physician, and Inez Perry, an astrologer, in their book "The Zodiac and the Salts of Salvation" published in 1932. They proposed that there is a relationship between the twelve astrological signs and the twelve biochemical cell salts and that each astrological sign corresponds to a particular cell salt.

According to their theory, an individual's astrological sign can give insights into their health needs. They can benefit from taking the corresponding cell salt to help balance their body's mineral levels. For example, a person born under the astrological sign of Aries may benefit from taking potassium phosphate (one of the cell salts) to support the nervous system and reduce stress and anxiety.

The 12 Cell Salts

1. Calcarea fluorica (Calcium fluoride) - Cancer

Foods: Turnips, Asparagus, Beets, Kelp, Garlic, Pineapple.

- It helps maintain the elasticity and strength of tissues, bones, and teeth.

- It also helps with hemorrhoids and hernia pain.

2. Calcarea phosphoric (Calcium phosphate) - Capricorn

Foods: Parsley, Beans, Beets, Carrots, Linseed Meal, Peanuts, Avocados.

- It promotes healthy bone and tissue growth, supports digestion, and aids nutrient absorption.

3. Calcarea sulphuric (Calcium sulfate) - Scorpio

Foods: Cauliflower, Lettuce, Cabbage, Turnips, Radishes, Onions, Celery, Brussels sprouts, Kohlrabi.

- It supports the immune system.

- It also helps the body fight infections and promotes healing.

- It treats skin disorders such as acne and Prevents sore throats and colds.

4. Ferrum phosphoricum (Iron phosphate) - Pisces

Foods: Raisins, Prunes, Plums, Grapes, Figs, Oranges, Spinach, Currants, Mushrooms, Dates, Beets, Wheat Bran, Lima Beans.

- It helps reduce inflammation.

- Supports immune system function and supports healthy blood circulation.

- Reduces fever.

- Accelerates healing.

- Reduces bleeding.

5. Kali Muriaticum (Potassium chloride) - Gemini

Foods: Radishes, Lentils, Carrots, Spinach, Asparagus, Sauerkraut.

- Aids in the breakdown of fibrin and mucus.

- It promotes healthy skin and hair.

- It also supports respiratory health.

- It treats infection, reduces swelling, and aids digestion.

6. Kali Phosphoricum (Potassium phosphate) - Aries

Foods: Parsley, Beans, Beets, Carrots, Linseed Meal, Peanuts, Avocados.

- It helps reduce stress and anxiety.

- It also supports the nervous system, promotes mental clarity and focus, and relieves headaches.

7. Kali Sulphuricum (Potassium sulphate) - Virgo

Foods: Cauliflower, Lettuce, Cabbage, Onions, Celery, Brussels sprouts, Tomatoes, Cucumbers.

- It supports healthy skin, Aids in detoxification.

- It also promotes healthy digestive function and balances metabolism.

- Conditions the pancreas.

8. Magnesia phosphoric (Magnesium phosphate) - Leo

Foods: Cauliflower, Cabbage, Asparagus, Almonds, Whole Wheat, Lemons, Limes, Oranges, Grapefruit, Figs, Gooseberries, Peaches, Cherries.

- It helps reduce cramps and spasms.

- It also supports healthy nerve function, aids nutrient absorption, and Increases pain and Relieves tension headaches.

9. Natrum Muriaticum (Sodium chloride) - Aquarius

Foods: Onions, Celery, Tomatoes, Almonds, Apples, Spinach, Peaches, Pecans, Lentils, Sauerkraut, Swiss chard

- It supports healthy fluid balance in the body and aids in nutrient absorption.

- It promotes healthy skin and hair and reduces water retention.

10. Natrum Phosphoricum (Sodium phosphate) - Libra

Foods: Brown Rice, Tomato juice, Citrus fruits and juices, Lentils, Vegetable Greens

- It supports healthy digestion and acid balance.

- It promotes healthy immune system function, aids nutrient absorption, neutralizes acidity, and treats arthritis.

11. Natrum Sulphuricum (Sodium sulphate)- Taurus

Foods: Cauliflower, Lettuce, Cabbage, Turnips, Radishes, Onions, Celery, Brussels sprouts, Kohlrabi.

- It supports healthy liver function and detoxification and aids in nutrient absorption.

- It promotes healthy digestion and cleanses the pancreas, kidneys, and liver. It also treats colds and flu.

12. Silicea (Silica) - Sagittarius

Foods: Endive, Barley, Oats, Raw Cabbage, Cucumber skins, Shredded Wheat, Rye and Whole Wheat products, Spinach, Peas, Carrots, Gooseberries, Strawberries

- It promotes healthy skin, hair, and nails.

- It supports healthy connective tissue, aids in absorbing minerals, conditions skin and connective tissue, and cleanses blood.

Amino Acids

Amino acids are the building blocks of proteins. They play a critical role in many physiological processes, including the growth and repair of tissues, the formation of enzymes and hormones, and the regulation of metabolism. There are 20 different types of amino acids, each with its unique chemical structure and function.

Several natural food sources contain a balanced mixture of all the essential and non-essential amino acids, also known as complete proteins. Some examples of such sources are:

- **Bee Pollen -** The number of amino acids in bee pollen can vary depending on various factors, such as the plant sources and location from where the pollen was collected. Typically, bee pollen contains all 20 of the amino acids that the human body requires for proper functioning. These include nine essential amino acids that the body cannot synthesize and must be obtained from the diet and 11 non-essential amino acids that the body can produce independently. The exact amounts of each amino acid in bee pollen can vary, but it generally contains a balanced mixture of all the essential and non-essential amino acids.

- **Quinoa -** Quinoa is a grain-like crop rich in protein and contains all the essential amino acids. It is also high in fiber, vitamins, and minerals.

- **Buckwheat -** Buckwheat is another grain-like crop that is a good source of complete protein. It is also high in fiber, antioxidants, and minerals.

- **Chia seeds -** Chia seeds are a type of seed that is rich in protein, fiber, omega-3 fatty acids, and antioxidants. They contain all the essential amino acids and are a good source of non-essential amino acids.

- **Hemp seeds -** Hemp seeds are a good source of complete protein and contain all the essential amino acids. They are also rich in healthy fats, fiber, and minerals.

- **Sea Moss -** Sea moss, also known as Irish moss or red seaweed, is commonly used as a food and dietary supplement. It contains various essential and non-essential amino acids necessary for human health. Some essential amino acids in sea moss include leucine, isoleucine, lysine, methionine, phenylalanine, threonine, tryptophan, and valine. The body cannot produce these amino acids, which must be obtained from the diet. In addition, sea moss also contains non-essential amino acids such as alanine, arginine, aspartic acid, cysteine, glutamic acid, glycine, histidine, proline, serine, and tyrosine. The exact amounts of each amino acid in sea moss can vary depending on the specific type of seaweed, growing conditions, and other factors; however, sea moss is generally considered a good source of protein and amino acids for human consumption.

- **Spirulina -** Spirulina is a type of blue-green algae rich in protein and contains all the essential amino acids. It is also a good source of vitamins, minerals, and antioxidants.

Vitamins

Vitamins are organic compounds that the body needs in small amounts to carry out specific functions, such as maintaining healthy skin, eyesight, and immune function. There are two main types of vitamins: fat-soluble and water-soluble. Fat-soluble vitamins, such as A, D, E, and K, are stored in the body's fatty tissues, while water-soluble vitamins, such as vitamin C and B vitamins, are not stored and must be obtained regularly through diet.

These 13 vitamins are essential for our body's normal growth, development, and overall health. Each vitamin plays a unique role in our body and is required in specific amounts through our diet or supplements.

- Vitamin A (Retinol)
- Vitamin B1 (Thiamine)
- Vitamin B2 (Riboflavin)
- Vitamin B3 (Niacin)
- Vitamin B5 (Pantothenic acid)
- Vitamin B6 (Pyridoxine)
- Vitamin B7 (Biotin)
- Vitamin B9 (Folate or folic acid)
- Vitamin B12 (Cobalamin)
- Vitamin C (Ascorbic acid)
- Vitamin D (Calciferol)
- Vitamin E (Tocopherol)
- Vitamin K (Phylloquinone or menaquinone)

Vitamin A (Retinol): Helps maintain healthy eyesight, skin, and immune function. Found in foods such as sweet potatoes, carrots, spinach, kale, collard greens, broccoli, apricots, cantaloupe, liver, eggs, and dairy products.

Vitamin B1 (Thiamine): Helps convert food into energy and supports the nervous system. Found in foods such as whole grains, fortified cereals, beans, nuts, seeds, pork, and yeast.

Vitamin B2 (Riboflavin): Helps convert food into energy and supports healthy skin and eyesight. Found in foods such as eggs, lean meats, mushrooms, spinach, almonds, and fortified cereals.

Vitamin B3 (Niacin): Helps convert food into energy and supports healthy skin, nerves, and digestion. Found in foods such as lean meats, poultry, fish, peanuts, whole grains, mushrooms, and fortified cereals.

Vitamin B5 (Pantothenic acid): Helps convert food into energy and supports healthy skin, hair, and nerves. It is found in foods such as meat, fish, and whole grains.

Vitamin B6 (Pyridoxine): Helps produce neurotransmitters that regulate mood and support healthy brain development. Found in foods such as poultry, fish, organ meats, potatoes, bananas, chickpeas, and fortified cereals.

Vitamin B7 (Biotin): Supports healthy skin, hair, and nails. Found in foods such as egg yolks, liver, nuts, seeds, sweet potatoes, and spinach.

Vitamin B9 (Folate or folic acid): Supports healthy fetal development during pregnancy and helps produce red blood cells. Found in foods such as leafy greens, asparagus, broccoli, beans, lentils, peas, and fortified cereals.

Vitamin B12 (Cobalamin): Helps produce red blood cells and supports healthy nerve function. It is found in foods such as meat, fish, poultry, eggs, milk, and fortified cereals.

Vitamin C (Ascorbic acid): Helps support a healthy immune system and aids in iron absorption. Found in foods such as citrus fruits, strawberries, kiwi, mango, pineapple, tomatoes, bell peppers, broccoli, and leafy greens.

Vitamin D (Calciferol): Helps the body absorb calcium for strong bones and teeth. Found in foods such as fatty fish, egg yolks, mushrooms exposed to UV light and fortified foods like milk, cereal, and orange juice, but *our body can also produce it when exposed to sunlight.*

Vitamin E (Tocopherol): It acts as an antioxidant that protects cells from damage and supports healthy skin and eyes. Found in foods such as nuts, seeds, vegetable oils, leafy greens, and fortified cereals.

Vitamin K (Phylloquinone or menaquinone): Helps with blood clotting and bone health. Found in foods such as leafy greens, broccoli, and vegetable oils, Brussels sprouts, asparagus.

- Vitamin K2, a subtype of vitamin K, is crucial for bone and heart health. It works by transporting calcium to the bones, which helps to prevent calcium from depositing in other tissues, such as the arteries. The specific subtype of vitamin K2 involved in this process is menaquinone-7 (MK-7).

• While natto is the richest dietary source of MK-7, some people may find its taste and texture unappealing. Other sources of MK-7 include certain types of cheese, miso, sauerkraut, kimchi, chicken, and eggs. Tempeh, a traditional Indonesian food made from fermented soybeans, is another rich source of MK-7.

• To make tempeh, soybeans are cooked, dehulled, and mixed with a starter culture of Rhizopus mold. The mixture is then left to ferment for 24-48 hours when the mold grows and binds the soybeans together into a cake-like form. Tempeh is a rich source of protein, fiber, and various vitamins and minerals, including vitamin K2. In addition to its nutritional benefits, tempeh is also considered a probiotic food, as the fermentation process promotes the growth of beneficial bacteria that can help support digestive health.

• By helping to transport calcium to the bones and teeth, vitamin K2 helps to maintain their structure and strength. It also plays a role in cardiovascular health by preventing calcium buildup in the arteries, which can lead to heart disease. Many individuals who find themselves taking calcium supplements later in life should look to incorporating more natural sources of Vitamin K2 into their diets, as that will help direct the calcium to where it needs to go.

Herbs And Mushrooms Supporting The 13 Essential Vitamins:

Vitamin A:

• Thyme

• Sage

• Oregano

• Parsley

• Basil

• Bay leaves

- Cilantro

- Rosemary

- Tarragon

- Lemongrass

- Reishi Mushroom

Vitamin C:

- Rose hips

- Thyme

- Sage

- Cilantro

- Peppermint

- Echinacea

- Lemon verbena

- Hibiscus

- Calendula

- Astragalus

Vitamin D:

- Alfalfa

- Stinging nettle

- Licorice root

- Burdock root

- Ginkgo biloba

- Horsetail

- Yellow dock

- Gotu Kola

- Calendula

- Dandelion root

Vitamin E:

- Basil

- Rosemary

- Sage

- Thyme

- Oregano

- Lavender

- Lemon balm

- Catnip

- Spearmint

- Chamomile

Vitamin K:

- Basil

- Parsley

- Thyme

- Sage

- Rosemary

- Oregano

- Bay leaves

- Lavender

- Lemon balm

- Peppermint

- Chaga Mushroom

- Reishi Mushroom

Thiamine (Vitamin B1):

- Basil

- Thyme

- Oregano

- Sage

- Bay leaves

- Dill

- Lemongrass

- Marjoram

- Lavender

- Catnip

- Reishi Mushroom

Riboflavin (Vitamin B2):

- Parsley

- Basil

- Thyme

- Sage

- Oregano

- Lemon balm

- Peppermint

- Spearmint

- Catnip

- Chamomile

- Lion's Mane Mushroom

Niacin (Vitamin B3):

- Chamomile

- Peppermint

- Lemon balm

- Lavender

- Catnip

- Passionflower

- Skullcap

- St. John's wort

- Valerian root

- Ginger root

Pantothenic Acid (Vitamin B5):

- Basil

- Thyme

- Sage

- Oregano

- Rosemary

- Lemongrass

- Marjoram

- Lavender

- Catnip

- Spearmint

- Chamomile

- Cordyceps Mushroom

- Reishi Mushroom

Pyridoxine (Vitamin B6):

- Basil

- Thyme

- Sage

- Oregano

- Rosemary

- Lavender

- Lemon balm

- Catnip

- Peppermint

- Chamomile

- Reishi Mushroom

Biotin (Vitamin B7):

- Nettle leaf

- Lavender

- Chamomile

- Calendula

- Red clover

- Burdock root

- Dandelion root

- Horsetail

- Yellow dock

- Gotu Kola

- Reishi Mushroom

- Lion's Mane Mushroom

Folate (Vitamin B9):

- Basil

- Parsley

- Thyme

- Sage

- Oregano

- Rosemary

- Lavender

- Lemon balm

- Peppermint

- Chamomile

- Reishi Mushroom

Cobalamin (Vitamin B12):

- Nettle leaf

- Red clover

- Burdock root

- Dandelion root

- Yellow dock

- Gotu Kola

- Milk thistle

- Hawthorn berry

- Ginkgo biloba

- Ginger root

- Reishi Mushroom

Parasites As A Root Cause Of Illness And Disease

"An understanding of parasite infestation and its treatment is essential for true vitality and strong immunity. Our observations indicate that more people are infected with worms and harmful micro-organisms than previously expected. If parasites are identified as a source of imbalance, **a parasite cleanse is in order before attempting to heal other aspects of the body.**" - Suzanne Shaw and Paul Pitchford.

No matter where you're at on your health and wellness journey, the longer we live, our responsibility is to be both accountable for our own health and conduct check-ups on ourselves; moreover, even when we're doing everything like working out, being mindful of a healthy diet, staying active in our lifestyle choices, and even laughing a lot, we still need to hit the body's 'reset 'button.

Excessively processed foods, breads, meats, dairy, sugars (non-fruit), fried foods, refined carbohydrates, and sodium get stored in our bodies throughout our lives.

We can easily understand the food-to-weight relationship that our bodies maintain, but we don't always consider the internal harm that excessive drinking, poor diet, and sedentary lifestyle choices inflict upon us. Even more, though tasty and delicious, these harmful foods don't always pass through our digestive systems properly, leaving behind waste and toxins that begin collecting on the walls of our intestines while clogging our liver and colon. This then begins not just to affect how our body absorbs the healthy nutrients it needs from food, but it also begins to cause issues with how our bodies are supposed to eliminate food, waste, and harmful toxins.

So now, ask yourself, "When was the last time I rewarded my various internal systems (respiratory, digestive, circulatory, nervous, etc.) with an all-natural, healthy reset?"

Seemingly, throughout the past couple of generations, the word 'detox 'has been tossed around rather carelessly; however, in its true meaning, a detox is a process or period in which one abstains from or rids the body of toxic and unhealthy substances.

This is important and applies to all, including seasoned individuals of health: Sometimes, after finding yourself making incredible leaps forward in your health journey, you may begin noticing certain habits, thoughts, and physical symptoms (bloating, depression, rashes, fatigue, light-headedness, etc.) are just not getting better. It's almost as if no matter what you do, something is hijacking your body to keep your energy and self in the past, though your actions and determined focus were clearly grounded in life's present and forward-moving cycles.

Though it is not likely that one has the common pinworm or roundworm (as unavoidable symptoms appear with these infestations), an individual could be living with one or multiple PARASITES in their body. The best thing a person can do is undergo an all-natural detox of their intestines and colon.

What are Parasites?

Before going further, let us discuss parasites for a moment:

1) A parasite is an organism that lives in another organism, called the host and often harms it. The parasite DEPENDS on it's host for survival.

2) The parasite uses the host's resources to fuel it's life cycle and maintain itself, often to the detriment of the host.

3) Parasites vary widely. Around 70 percent are not visible to the human eye, such as the malarial parasite, yet some worm parasites can reach over 30 meters in length!

4) Parasites are not a disease, but they can spread diseases! Also - different parasites have different harmful effects on the human body.

Parasites, unlike predators, are usually much smaller than their host and reproduce faster.

Without a host, a parasite cannot live, grow and multiply.

Types of Parasites

There are three types of parasites: Ectoparasites, Protozoa, Helminths (worms)

We've become familiar with parasites outside the body, known as Ectoparasites, like fleas, ticks, bedbugs, body lice, crab lice, scabies, and head lice; however, protozoa and worms (helminth organisms) can affect humans and animals from INSIDE the body. Though we have a minimal number of options for over-the-counter (OTC) medication to help with pinworms and roundworms, there are MANY other types of worms, protozoa, and their parasitic infections that cause harm to our human bodies, including Anisakiasis, Racoon Roundworm, Clonorchiasis, Ddioctophyme Renalis Infection, Diphyllobothriasis Tapeworm, Guinea Worm, Hookworm, Hymenolepiasis, Echinococcosis Tape Worm, Enterobiasis Pinworm, Fasciolosis

Liver Fluke, Fasciolopsiasis Intestinal Fluke, Gnathostomiasis, Loa Loa Filariasis, Mansonellosis, Onchocerca Volvulus, Lung Fluke, Entamoeba Histolytica, Trypanosoma, Acanthamoebiasis, Babesiosis, Balantidiasis, Blastocystosis, Coccidiosis and more!

Research has proven that there is no credible way of estimating how many parasitic protozoa, fungi, bacteria, and viruses exist. According to a study published in the National Academy of Sciences, we can estimate that there are between 75,000 and 300,000 worm/helminth species parasitizing vertebrates.

Parasitic Locations and Symptoms

When you have a parasitic infestation, you are the host. Then, the parasite is doing everything in its power to operate your body as if it were a car, driving you to achieve what it wants. Let us take this moment to remember that we are energetic beings who are constantly responding to stimuli and impulses. For this reason, identifying the bodily location of the parasite helps determine the actions it is influencing and forcing the body to make.

Parasites enter the body, and like a computer with malware or a virus, they are slowly draining the processing power and life-force of the body; moreover, similar to computer malware that may come from clicking a link and/or opening an email, website or file, parasites can come from ex-partners, pets, public surfaces and foods that we engage with. The trouble is that when we don't routinely eliminate parasites, we can be living with them for years and even the entirety of our lives, without realizing that we have an internal infestation. Individuals who have done detoxes, therapy and/or practice many self-care techniques may still wonder why they can't seem to lose those last few pounds, stop thinking of an ex and/or let go of childhood trauma, and unfortunately, it may be because of un-eliminated parasites that entered their body during those encounters. In traditional folk medicine, here are the locations and actions that parasites are said to infest.

Prostate or Womb = Increased sexual drive thereby finding ourselves in actions that release too much of our bodily fluids.

Small Intestine = Eat Sweets

Large Intestine = Eating Foods that Promote Constipation

Kidneys = Salty Foods

Lungs - Force Cough or Pick Up Something to Smoke

Liver = Irritable/Angry. Blood boils in the liver

Head = Force you to stop listening to gut intuition

Eyes = Disrupts your focus balance. It forces you not to see clearly.

Since parasites can pass on various conditions and infections, symptoms are sometimes hard to predict. Even when there are no symptoms or if symptoms often appear long after the infection, the parasite can still be transmitted to another person who may develop symptoms. Symptoms may include:

• Recurring skin bumps or rashes

• Weight loss, increased appetite or both

• Abdominal pain, diarrhea and vomiting

• Sleeping problems

• Anemia

• Aches and pains

• Allergies

• Weakness and general feeling unwell

• Fever

Detoxing Your Body of Harmful Parasites

These recommendations are ideal for anyone with apparent symptoms associated with parasites. In addition to those who consume meat, fish, and poultry, have pets, touch bare surfaces, and walk surfaces with bare feet, in agreement with other leading herbal practitioners, a parasite purge program 'should also be followed by virtually everyone with lingering illnesses or degenerative conditions (e.g., cancer, arthritis, AIDS, chronic fatigue syndromes, alcoholism, etc.). Parasitic pathogens nearly ALWAYS play a role in the etiology (the cause, set of causes, or manner of causation of a disease or condition) of degeneration.'

As we purge parasites, we must also remember that they too have energetic attachments and entanglements. The process of parasitic elimination is very much a 'cord cutting ceremony', and for this reason, parties on the other end who were feeding and/or robbing nourishment from the body are now VERY unhappy. This is why even though we are doing the work for ourselves, internally and externally, other entities (parasites, parasitic individuals who drain your energy/energy vampires, abusive partners, others who are proud to live their unhealthiest lives with you, etc) will do their best to throw you off track and/or try to have you fallback into old ways. Their survival is dependent upon YOU, at your own peril!

In the universe, a powerful cosmic reset happens that affects everyone on the planet, and yet, many of us are completely unaware; moreover, it is during these resets that we actually find that the planet and universe are aligned to support us in cleansing the body of parasites.

Many people would be surprised to learn that even in the Farmer's Almanac, the ancestral understanding that parasites are most active during full moons is stated multiple times, and it is also indicated that this is the best time to kill/eliminate/purge parasites from unwanted places like the garden and body. With our planetary revolution being a 360 degree cycle, the 180 degree points indicate the moments that Earth is halfway through its approximate 365-day yearly cycle, and 14 days before Earth reaches its halfway points, we have full moons and the beginnings of new seasons, with both the Winter and Summer Solstices.

Did you know that people travel from all over the world to be at the ancient monument Stonehenge for the solstices? We have now come to appreciate and know this monument to be just as profound as the pyramids of Egypt, in its alignment with our celestial, cosmic clock, and in these gatherings where individuals are honoring the profound cosmic alignment, how many are also doing the work to honor their internal clock aka circadian rhythm, to best prepare for the seasons ahead?

14 days after the solstices, we encounter what's known as the Solar Aphelion and Solar Perihelion— the days in which our planet is the farthest and closest to the sun during the year; moreover, in the United States of America, we have been so distracted with the preparation, celebration and overconsumption of holiday consumerism, we're completely disassociated from these universals energies.

Think about it, despite the astronomical significance of these events, in the USA, most of us are too busy burdening our body and health with everything New Year's Eve and Fourth of July that we are doing the very opposite of what these cosmic events are telling us to do…which is: Rest, reset, be gracious, honor the light, detox, let go and prepare for the seasons ahead. Remember: We are seasonal beings of the natural world, not beings meant for a "9 to 5 + overtime = Burnout" existence.

So consider treating yourself to this birthright, ancestral practice that is truly aligned with the rhythms, energy, frequency and vibrations of our planet. Remember: Parasite Cleanse during the solstices, and 14 days later, begin an all-natural, herbal cellular detox, on/around the Solar Perihelion and/or Aphelion.

Traditional Herbs Used to Eliminate Parasites

Here is a list of herbs known to help support intestinal health that you can incorporate into your wellness routine!

- Pumpkin Seed
- Black Walnut Hull
- Wormwood
- Celery Seed
- Garlic
- Cloves
- Bitter Melon
- Pau d'Arco
- Diatomaceous Earth

Before beginning a reset with the **Circadian360 Cellular Detox Tea**, one should complete a **Circadian360 Parasite Cleanse** first!

Excessive Congestion, Mucus, And Inflammation As Root Causes Of Illness and Disease

If the body is a car, the quality of fuel that one puts inside certainly matters. Just as we wash our cars to keep them clean, how often and when we get a checkup (self-assessment), oil change (detox), and heavy service work (surgery) matters too.

We must remember that food is meant to be our cellular energy! It is how we fuel our light body. All food is eventually converted into glucose (sugar) in the body, which serves as a source of cellular energy, particularly for the brain. The speed at which food is converted to sugar and enters the bloodstream is called the glycemic index(GI), measuring how quickly the carbohydrates in a particular food raise blood sugar levels.

In *The Big Picture*, we broke down the fact that even our foods have aligned frequencies, affected and relying upon the rhythms of the sun, highlighting the importance of raw foods. When it comes to processed foods, the term "processed" generally refers to foods that have undergone various forms of manufacturing or refinement. These foods often contain added sugars, unhealthy fats, and other additives. Food processing can remove or alter its natural fiber content, affecting how quickly the body breaks down and absorbs carbohydrates.

Consuming processed foods, especially those with high glycemic indexes, can cause a rapid increase in blood sugar levels. This can stress the pancreas, producing insulin to regulate blood sugar levels. If the pancreas cannot produce enough insulin to compensate for the rapid spike in blood sugar, it can lead to various health issues, including insulin resistance and type 2 diabetes.

On the other hand, raw foods, such as fruits, vegetables, and whole grains, typically have a lower glycemic index because they contain more natural fiber and are digested more slowly. The slower digestion process allows for a more gradual release of glucose into the bloodstream, which helps maintain stable blood sugar levels and provides sustained energy. This emphasis on consuming raw foods is beneficial for managing blood sugar levels and addressing another overlooked factor in overall health: **congestion**.

Congestion is often overlooked as a root cause of illness and disease. It can manifest in different body areas and lead to various health conditions. For example, lung congestion can lead to chronic obstructive pulmonary disease (COPD), while circulatory congestion can lead to heart disease and stroke. Congestion occurs when there is an accumulation of fluids, waste, and toxins in the body. It can be caused by poor dietary choices, lack of exercise, and exposure to environmental toxins.

Inflammation is closely related to congestion. Congestion can trigger an inflammatory response in the body as the immune system tries to remove the buildup of waste and toxins. Inflammation is a natural response of the body's immune system to injury or infection. It is a complex process that involves releasing certain chemicals, such as cytokines and prostaglandins, which help increase blood flow to the affected area, activate immune cells to fight off foreign invaders, like bacteria or viruses, and repair damaged tissue. While inflammation is a crucial part of the healing process, chronic inflammation can lead to various health problems, such as cardiovascular disease, arthritis, and cancer. Various factors, including poor diet, lack of exercise, stress, exposure to toxins, and chronic infections can trigger it.

Mucus is a viscous substance produced by mucous membranes in the body that serves as a protective layer in various body parts, such as the respiratory tract, gastrointestinal tract, and reproductive system; however, excessive mucus production can indicate inflammation or other health issues because it is the body's response to irritation or infection. Chronic inflammation, in particular, has been linked to many chronic diseases, including heart disease, diabetes, arthritis, and cancer.

Certain dietary factors have been shown to increase mucus production in the body.

For example, when consumed in excess, starch can contribute to mucus production in the body by leading to an overgrowth of certain types of bacteria in the gut that can produce mucus as a byproduct. Meat consumption has also been shown to increase mucus production, likely due to the high levels of protein and fat in meat that can increase the production of mucus-producing cells in the body. More evidence is showing that many individuals should reconsider their dairy consumption.

Did you know that according to the National Institutes of Health (NIH), approximately 65-75% of African Americans have some degree of lactose intolerance? This means that some individuals are unable to digest lactose, a sugar found in milk and dairy products, due to a deficiency of the enzyme lactase. Nevertheless, how can we be lactose intolerant if we are supposed to be breastfed by our mothers upon birth?

As people age, lactase production, the enzyme responsible for breaking down lactose, tends to decrease. Lactase is typically most abundant during infancy and childhood when milk is a primary source of nutrition; however, as individuals mature and their diets diversify, the need for lactase production decreases, leading to a decline in production. Beyond this, some ethnic groups are genetically predisposed to reduce their lactase activity after infancy naturally. This is known as primary lactose intolerance and is more common in people of East Asian, African, Hispanic, and Native American descent. In these cases, lactose intolerance may be more likely to develop at a younger age.

It isn't typically until the individual has developed past infancy that the symptoms of lactose intolerance manifest; moreover, more studies are being revealed that show the detrimental harm that dairy products potentially can have when consumed by some especially individuals of color.

80% of African American women will develop fibroids at some point in their lifetime. In recent years, the correlation between specific dietary and lifestyle factors and the development of fibroids in women has garnered increased attention. Among the most concerning endocrine disruptors associated with fibroid development are substances found in soy and dairy products and specific hair care products such as chemical straighteners. Particularly among women of color, these disruptors tend to elevate estrogen levels.

Soy, a widely popular plant-based protein source often consumed as an alternative to animal products, contains phytoestrogens. These compounds can imitate the effects of estrogen in the body. This can pose problems for women since elevated estrogen levels have been linked to a heightened risk of fibroid development; moreover, soy has been found to stimulate mucus production in the body, potentially leading to respiratory complications and other health concerns.

On the other hand, dairy products contain a protein called casein linked to the development of fibroids. Casein is difficult for the body to digest and can lead to inflammation, contributing to the development of fibroids.

Did you catch that?

Remember - according to the National Institutes of Health (NIH), approximately 65-75% of African Americans have some degree of lactose intolerance. It just SO HAPPENS that 80% of ALL African American women will develop fibroids caused by excessive estrogen from excessive consumption of products, including dairy and soy.

This is significant to acknowledge because when you consider that BUTTER IS DAIRY, even when we are commonly promoting healthy recipes that use butter and salt to sauté vegetables, individuals unknowingly STILL silently kill themselves through hypertension and chronic inflammation while ramping up their estrogen production; moreover, some evidence suggests that excessive consumption of seed oils, particularly those high in omega-6 fatty acids, may impact estrogen production and hormonal balance!

Omega-6 fatty acids are essential fats in various seed oils such as corn, soybean, sunflower, cottonseed, grapeseed, peanut, sesame, and safflower. While omega-6 fatty acids are necessary for normal bodily functions, excessive consumption of these fats, especially when not balanced with omega-3 fatty acids, may lead to an imbalance in the omega-6 to omega-3 ratio. Some studies have suggested that a high omega-6 to omega-3 ratio may promote inflammation and disrupt hormonal balance, including estrogen levels.

Chronic inflammation and hormonal imbalances have been associated with various health issues.

Another factor linked to the development of fibroids in women is using certain hair care products, particularly chemical straighteners. These products often contain ingredients like formaldehyde, disrupting the body's hormone balance and increasing the risk of developing fibroids. Many of these products are also known to increase mucus production in the body, leading to other health issues.

It is important for women, particularly women of color, to be aware of these risks and to make informed choices about their diet, lifestyle, and personal care products. Reducing or eliminating soy and dairy products from your diet and avoiding chemical hair straighteners and other harmful hair care products can greatly reduce your risk of developing fibroids and other health issues.

Research has shown a strong link between estrogen and fibroids, and lifestyle factors like diet and personal care products can significantly affect hormone balance. In one study, **women who consumed more than one serving of dairy products per day were found to have a 30% increased risk of developing fibroids compared to women who consumed less than one serving per day**. *Additionally, a study conducted in 2012 found that women who used hair relaxers were more likely to develop fibroids than women who did not use these products.*

Excessive congestion, mucus, and inflammation often stem from deep emotional bonds, habits, and traumas that are tied to the culprits harming our health, as mentioned above. These factors must be addressed during an individual's healing journey. Otherwise, one may have never-ending love/hate cycles and relationships with certain unhealthy foods, activities, and environments. The tricky part is that some unhealthy attachments were forged during infancy, and this goes back to when we discussed epigenetic's earlier in this book, in relation to breaking the generational curses that are within our control.

When we look at the protein casein inside dairy products, we find that it plays a crucial role in providing essential amino acids and nutrients to support the growth and development of young mammals, but not all mammal milk is equal!

In general, cow milk's casein content is higher than human milk's. Cow milk typically contains around 2.5-3.5 grams of casein per 100 milliliters, whereas human milk contains about 0.2-0.4 grams per 100 milliliters; therefore, cow milk has approximately 6-15 times more casein than human milk.

The trouble with this is that casein also plays a role in bonding between a calf and it's mother. When a calf consumes milk, the casein proteins are broken down into smaller peptides during digestion. One of these peptides is called casomorphin, an **opioid-like substance**.

Casomorphin has been found to have a calming effect on the calf and can promote a sense of contentment and attachment. This bonding process is important for the calf's emotional well-being and social development.

So when the human baby is most vulnerable and dependent upon the mother and/or other sources for food, security, shelter, support, love, respect, understanding, laughter, joy, rest, comfort, and soothing, they are given a bottle of formula, animal-derived milk and/or milk-based products every time they cry. The baby unknowingly associates comfort, contentment, resolution, peace, understanding, communication, love, acceptance, support, and respect with unhealthy foods and/or the methods by which said foods are consumed.

There is a reason ice cream, pizza, cake, butter, cheesecake, mac and cheese, cookies, grilled cheese sandwiches, and other popular dairy-heavy foods are amongst our favorite comfort foods! Since birth, many of us have been raised to lean on those foods for ALL occasions.

As you can guess, casein can stimulate mucus production and increase inflammation, leading to further mucus accumulation. Sugar consumption has also been shown to increase mucus production in the body by contributing to inflammation and an overgrowth of harmful bacteria in the gut that can produce mucus. Acidic foods can particularly damage the mucous membrane, causing an imbalance in the body's pH levels and leading to inflammation. Inflammation can then lead to an overproduction of mucus, further irritating and damaging the mucous membrane.

Supporting the health of the mucous membrane and minimizing mucus production can be achieved by adopting a diet rich in fruits, vegetables, and whole grains. This dietary choice helps alkalize the body and reduces inflammation.

Alkalizing The Body

When someone refers to the act of "helping to alkalize the body," they typically are talking about the body's pH balance.

The pH scale measures the acidity or alkalinity of a substance and ranges from 0 to 14. A pH of 7 is considered neutral, values below 7 are acidic, and values above 7 are alkaline or basic. This is the same pH scale many of us explored using the Litmus test's color-changing paper strips in science classes.

Championed by the late holistic health advocate Dr. Sebi through his teachings of the African Bio-Mineral Diet, proponents of alkalizing the body believe that maintaining a slightly alkaline pH level (around 7.35 to 7.45) benefits overall health and well-being. They claim an alkaline environment can help prevent or mitigate various health conditions, including inflammation, digestive disorders, and cancer. To support alkalization, advocates often recommend consuming certain foods and beverages considered alkaline-forming, such as fruits, vegetables, nuts, seeds, and certain types of water. These foods are believed to help counteract the acidic byproducts of metabolism and create a more alkaline state in the body; however, the human body has complex mechanisms to regulate its pH levels within a narrow range and does so quite effectively. Many promote the idea that the body has a single pH level, but this is far from the truth! The pH of different body parts, such as the blood, digestive system, and urine, can vary, and the body maintains the necessary pH balance for proper functioning.

This is why a healthy diet with high-frequency and alkalizing foods is ideal for proper body functioning, helping to reduce excessive congestion, mucus, and inflammation. Drinking plenty of water can also help to flush toxins from the body and keep the mucous membrane hydrated. Additionally, reducing stress and getting enough rest and exercise can help to support overall immune function and maintain the health of the mucous membrane.

By following the circadian rhythm's schedule for intermittent fasting and incorporating suggested herbs, mushrooms, astringent fruits, and lemon/lime-infused water, along with adopting a plant-based diet, you can help relieve congestion and inflammation, lower blood pressure and blood sugar levels, and improve overall health in many ways.

Face Mapping

Circadian360's Face Mapping

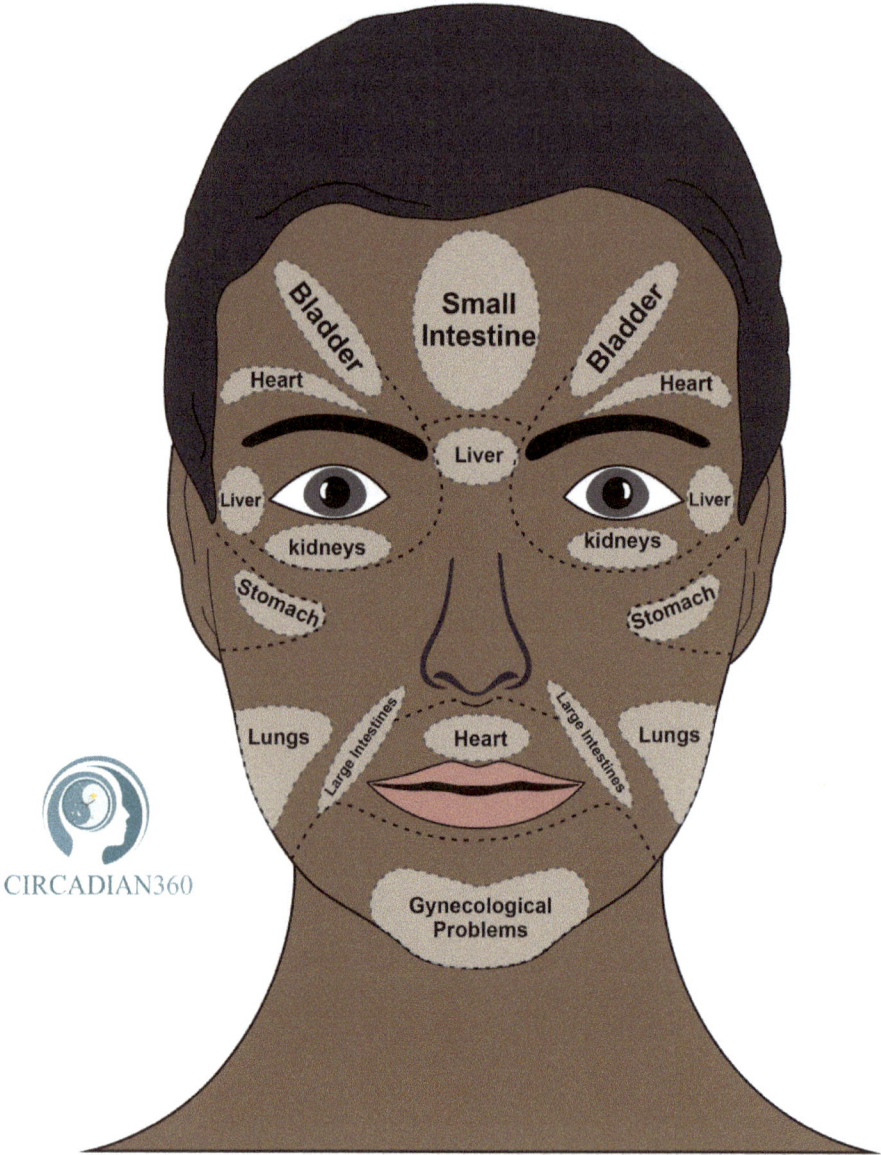

Face Mapping operates on the understanding that our external appearance, including the condition of our skin, reflects the state of our internal health and well-being.

Circadian360's Faces of Overconsumption

DAIRY

- Swollen eyelids
- Under eye bags
- Dark circles under the eye
- Acne all over the face
- Pale cheeks
- Concentrated spots on the chin

Eyelids puffy and swollen

Dark circles and bags under the eyes

Widespread acne and spots

Very pale cheeks

ALCOHOL

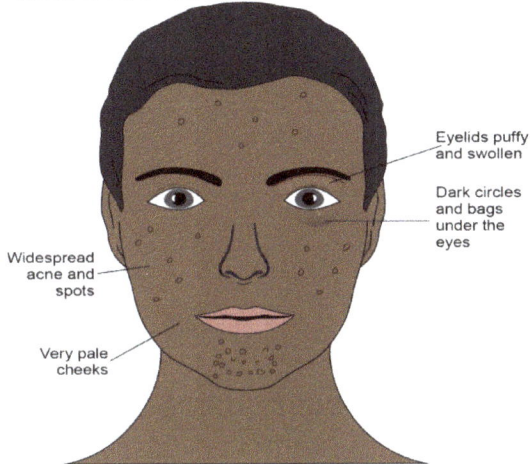

- Deep nasolabial folds
- Pronounced lines and deep furrows between the brows
- Saggy eyelids
- Fine lines and wrinkles under the eyes
- Dehydrated skin with soft feathery lines across the cheeks
- Enlarged pores
- Red skin tone

Deep lines or spots between the eyes

Droppy eyelids

Enlarged pores under eyes

Dehydrated skin with fine feathery lines across the cheeks

Fine Lines and wrinkles under the eyes

Redish tone to the skin

Deep nasolabial folds

GLUTEN

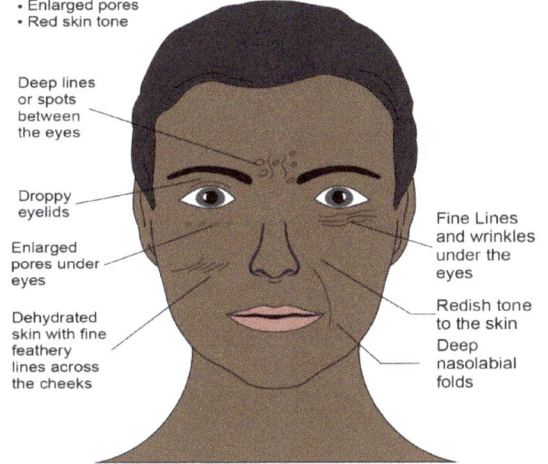

- Breakouts on the forehead
- Redness or red spots on the cheeks
- Dark patches or redness on the chin
- Puffy cheeks

Spots on forehead

Spots on cheeks

Puffy and red cheeks

Spots on the chin

Dark patches on the chin

SUGAR

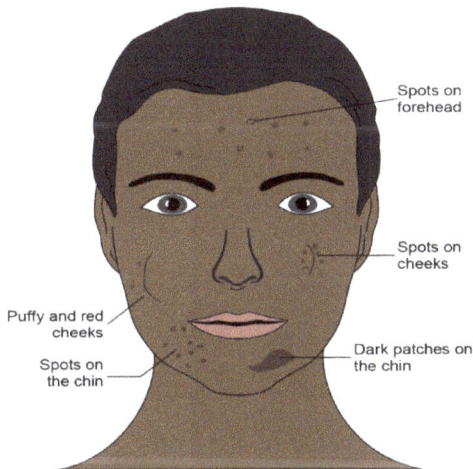

- Sagging skin under the eyes
- Deep lines and wrinkles on the upper forehead
- Pustular/ Cystic acne all over the face
- A gaunt look to the face
- Thinning of the skin
- Dark greyish or pasty white skin

Deep furrows on the upper forehead

Saggy under the eyes

A greyish white paled look to the skin

Thinning of the skin

Pustular spots all over the face

Hollow and gaunt look to the skin

CIRCADIAN360

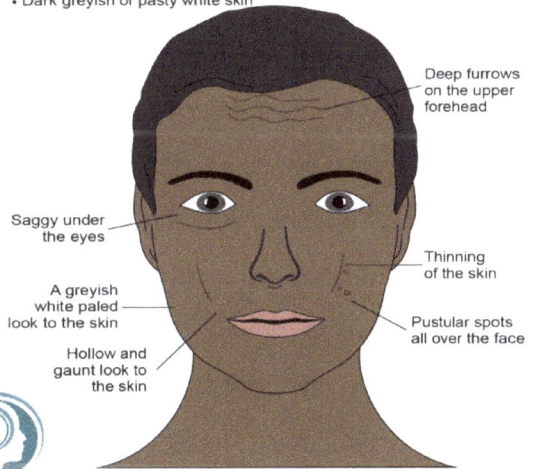

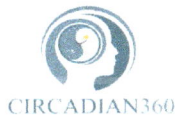

Considering the intricate network of meridians and the body's self-regulating capacity, it becomes apparent that an imbalance in the digestive system can manifest as skin issues, emphasizing the interconnectedness of our organs. Our skin is the largest external organ, constituting the canvas of our physicality. It follows that issues surfacing on the skin might signify internal imbalances demanding attention for holistic healing and optimal health. Pimples, rashes, or skin color/tone alterations can manifest underlying internal problems.

Delving deeper, through Traditional Chinese Medicine and other cultures, we find that the face represents a microcosm that unveils the body's inner workings. Just as acupuncture practitioners use fine needles to help stimulate life force/energy/Qi flow through meridian lines and points, face mapping reveals specific connections between facial areas and internal organs.

Mental Health

Meditation And The Third Eye/Pineal Gland

Shrouded in centuries of mystery and often called the "third eye," the pineal gland has captured the imagination of seekers, mystics, and scholars alike. This small, pinecone-shaped gland nestled deep within the brain has been attributed with remarkable functions that extend far beyond its tiny size. While some notions about the pineal gland may border on speculation, a wealth of scientific and cultural context invites us to explore its intriguing potential.

While traditional medical teachings might label it simply as a vestige of evolution that has diminished in function over time, emerging scientific understanding points to its significance in regulating the body's internal clock. At the heart of this intricate timekeeping is the suprachiasmatic nucleus (SCN), a cluster of cells within the brain's hypothalamus. The SCN acts as the master conductor of the body's circadian rhythms, governing the ebb and flow of biological processes over a 24-hour cycle.

The pineal gland's role in this chronobiological symphony is intimately tied to its ability to produce the hormone melatonin. This hormone is intricately linked to the sleep-wake cycle, with its production and release influenced by the SCN's signals in response to changes in light and darkness. As daylight fades, the SCN sends signals that prompt the pineal gland to ramp up melatonin production, inducing a sense of drowsiness and preparing the body for rest. Conversely, as morning light emerges, melatonin production decreases, helping to awaken the body and kick-start daily activities.

The pineal gland has been central in spiritual and cultural symbolism throughout history. From the eye of Horus in ancient Egypt to the notion of it being your inner seat to the "Door of Paradise," the gland has woven itself into the fabric of human understanding. Its depiction as a pineapple, laden with meaning in the Catholic and Masonic traditions, speaks to its significance.

The mysterious pineal gland is an orchestrator of complex biochemical processes that synchronizes our biological rhythms with the external world. The intricate dance between the pineal gland, the SCN, and the changing light patterns underscores the fascinating interplay between our internal biology and the external environment. As science continues to delve into the depths of this special relationship, we uncover layers of insight into how our bodies align with the rhythm of life itself.

The Third Eye and Multidimensional Connections

The concept of the pineal gland as the "third eye" is emblematic of its perceived role as a gateway to other dimensions of reality. This notion echoes across cultures, from the Eastern philosophies that embrace the Ajna chakra to the esoteric traditions that symbolize visionary insight. Whether one speaks of astral journeys, heightened intuition, or encounters with beings from other dimensions, the pineal gland is said to facilitate experiences that transcend the limits of our physical senses.

The Chemical Symphony: DMT and Altered States

The pineal gland's role in altered states of consciousness has been linked to DMT (dimethyltryptamine), often called the "spirit molecule." This compound is known for its hallucinogenic properties and occurrence in dreams and near-death experiences.

During intense dreaming, the pineal gland releases DMT, which might explain dreams' vivid and sometimes surreal nature; furthermore, DMT has also been associated with mystical experiences and inter-dimensional journeys, offering glimpses into realms beyond our everyday ordinary perception.

The Calcification of the Pineal Gland

Pineal gland calcification is a natural process that tends to increase with age. It involves the build up of calcium phosphate crystals in the pineal tissue.

The exact cause of pineal gland calcification is not fully understood yet; however, research suggests that factors such as genetics, lifestyle factors such as diet, exposure to certain environmental toxins, and even exposure to sunlight may play a role in the rate of pineal gland calcification.

Studies have shown significant differences in the degree of pineal gland calcification among individuals. Some people may have a relatively low degree of calcification, even in old age, while others may have a more heavily calcified pineal gland; moreover, some studies have suggested possible links between increased pineal gland calcification and Alzheimer's disease and mood disorders.

Additional research has suggested that dietary factors, such as a high fluoride intake or inadequate intake of certain minerals like magnesium, may influence the rate of pineal gland calcification. As the pineal gland is sensitive to light, and exposure to natural sunlight during the day and darkness at night helps regulate its melatonin production, disruptions in the light-dark cycle, such as shift work or excessive exposure to artificial light at night, may affect the pineal gland's function and increase the chances for pineal gland calcification. I wouldn't be surprised if we found that younger individuals are developing calcium deposits on their pineal gland, due to their generation's early adoption of certain lifestyle factors that are now being linked to potentially increasing the gland's calcification.

Awakening The Inner Temple: Meditation And Spiritual Practices

For those seeking to tap into the potential of the pineal gland, meditation offers a key.

This practice, found across spiritual traditions, is thought to activate and balance the energy centers, including the third eye. By quieting the mind and focusing awareness, meditation creates a conducive environment for exploring altered states of consciousness and connecting with the deeper dimensions of being.

Here's a list of meditative practices and mental health activities that are believed to promote the health and stimulation of the pineal gland:

Meditation: Regular meditation, especially techniques focusing on the third eye (such as Ajna chakra meditation), can help activate and balance the pineal gland. Visualization practices and guided meditations that involve imagining light entering the third eye can be beneficial.

Breath Work: Deep, rhythmic breathing exercises, in which you consciously control your breath, can help increase oxygen flow to the brain and support pineal gland health.

Mindfulness: Practicing mindfulness and staying present at the moment can reduce stress and improve overall brain function, potentially benefiting the pineal gland. The Circadian360 Mindfulness & Manifestations Workbook offers encouragement and guidance for you, in this this exploration.

Yoga: Certain yoga poses, like a child's pose and forward bends, can stimulate the third eye area and promote blood flow to the brain.

Sungazing: Gazing at the rising or setting sun during safe hours (only during the first and last hour of sunlight) is believed to stimulate the pineal gland due to the light's connection with the gland's melatonin regulation.

Sound Healing: Listening to specific frequencies or binaural beats corresponding to the pineal gland's resonance can encourage activation. Some believe that 432 Hz and 936 Hz frequencies are particularly beneficial.

Essential Oils: Certain essential oils, like frankincense and sandalwood, are believed to support pineal gland health. Diffusing these oils during meditation or relaxation can potentially have a positive effect.

Avoiding Fluoride: Reducing fluoride exposure, often found in tap water and toothpaste, supports pineal gland health as fluoride can accumulate in the gland and hinder its function.

Natural Foods: Consuming foods rich in antioxidants, such as dark leafy greens, walnuts, berries, and raw cacao, can provide nutrients that support overall brain health, potentially benefiting the pineal gland.

Intermittent Fasting: Some believe intermittent fasting may help regulate hormones and improve pineal gland function, especially at night.

Reducing Artificial Blue Light Exposure: Reducing screen time, especially before bedtime, can support the production of melatonin, which the pineal gland regulates.

Nature Connection: Spending time in nature, especially barefoot, can help balance your body's energy and connect you with the Earth's natural frequencies, potentially benefiting the pineal gland.

Dream Journaling: Keeping a dream journal can encourage better dream recall, potentially enhancing your connection with the subconscious mind and the pineal gland's role in dreaming.

Positive Affirmations: Repeating positive affirmations related to intuition, insight, and spiritual growth can help shift your focus toward activating the pineal gland.

While the pineal gland's precise functions and role in connecting with other dimensions remain subjects of ongoing research and contemplation, its cultural and historical significance cannot be denied. From ancient symbolism to modern scientific curiosity, the pineal gland continues to captivate minds and hearts alike.

The pineal gland invites us to explore the realms beyond the physical, journey within ourselves, and perhaps uncover the hidden potential within each of us.

Physical Health

The Science of "Hope Molecules": How Exercise Enhances Mental Health

Recent discoveries have unveiled a fascinating link between exercise and the release of what are now being referred to as "**hope molecules.**" These molecules, including proteins such as myokines, can significantly impact mood, strength, and overall mental health. In this section, we'll get into the groundbreaking concept of "hope molecules," shedding light on how exercise contributes to mental wellness.

Hope Molecules

The notion of "hope molecules" stems from the understanding that our bodies produce specific proteins that profoundly impact the brain in response to exercise. One key category of these molecules is myokines, which are released when muscles contract during physical activity. Myokines have gained attention for their potential to promote mental health and resilience.

The Role of Myokines

Myokines are not only responsible for the physiological benefits of exercise but also hold the key to enhancing mental well-being:

1. Brain-Boosting Effects: Myokines have been found to cross the blood-brain barrier and influence brain function, leading to improved mood, cognitive function, and emotional regulation.

2. Neurogenesis: Exercise-induced myokines can stimulate the growth of new brain cells, particularly in areas associated with memory and emotional processing.

3. Reducing Inflammation: Certain myokines possess anti-inflammatory properties, which are significant as chronic inflammation is linked to mental health disorders.

Mood Enhancement through Exercise

Regular physical activity has a profound impact on mood, and the presence of "hope molecules" plays a significant role:

1. Endorphins and Beyond: Beyond the well-known endorphins, myokines add another layer to the mood-boosting effects of exercise, promoting happiness and well-being.

2. Stress Reduction: Myokines reduce stress hormones and encourage relaxation, which can mitigate the effects of anxiety and stress.

Strength, Resilience, and Mental Health

The benefits of "hope molecules" extend to building mental resilience and strength:

1. Psychological Resilience: Exercise-induced myokines foster psychological resilience, enabling individuals to cope better with life's challenges and bounce back from adversity.

2. Confidence and Self-Efficacy: The positive impact of exercise on mental health contributes to increased confidence and self-efficacy, empowering individuals to overcome obstacles.

Incorporating Exercise for Mental Wellness

The concept of "hope molecules" highlights the importance of integrating regular exercise into a holistic approach to mental health:

1. A Balanced Routine: Engaging in various forms of exercise, from aerobic activities and calisthenics to strength training, can maximize the release of beneficial myokines.

2. Consistency Matters: Consistent exercise routines are essential for the sustained release of "hope molecules" and the associated mental health benefits.

3. Mind-Body Connection: Combining physical activity with mindfulness techniques such as yoga or meditation can amplify the effects on mental well-being.

Nurturing Mitochondrial Health: Unveiling the Cellular Powerhouses

In the intricate tapestry of human health, the realm of mitochondria is often overlooked but profoundly influential. These microscopic powerhouses, residing within our cells, hold the key to vitality, longevity, metabolism, and even the reduction of oxidative stress; however, very few of us are heeding the call to care for these vital energy producers amidst our modern-day flurry of health pursuits.

Mitochondria: The Engine of Life

Recall the lessons from biology class where mitochondria were introduced as the cell's powerhouse. It's a fitting description, as these remarkable structures generate a staggering 90% of the body's energy, yet their role transcends mere energy production. The health of your mitochondria weaves a tapestry of well-being, and conversely, unhealthy mitochondria cast shadows of ill health.

The Journey to Optimized Mitochondrial Health

1. Mitigating Artificial Blue Light Exposure: Artificial blue light, emitted from

screens and lightbulbs, disrupts mitochondrial harmony. This seemingly innocuous light acts as a toxin, increasing oxidative stress that undermines mitochondrial function. Limiting your exposure, especially before bedtime, protects your cellular powerhouses.

2. Nourishing with Essential Nutrients: Mitochondria crave a palette of nutrients for optimal function. Acetyl L-carnitine, magnesium, lipoic acid, omega-3s, B vitamins, vitamin E, selenium, and CoQ10 are their lifeblood. Seek these nutrients from whole food sources to support the mitochondrial symphony.

3. Bathing in Red Light: Red light emerges as a healing balm for your mitochondria. Embrace the natural rays of sunrise and sunset, allowing sunlight to caress your skin. Alternatively, invite a red light device into your home to bathe your cells in this regenerative hue.

4. Minimizing Oxidative Stress: Oxidative stress, the antagonist of mitochondrial health, undermines their structure and function. Say no to seed oils like canola, safflower, and sunflower. Opt for oils like olive, ghee, butter, and coconut that bestow a shield of protection upon your mitochondria. Also minimize toxin exposure to protect the sanctity of these cellular engines.

5. Embracing Antioxidants: In the battle against oxidative stress, antioxidants emerge as valiant defenders. Foods like citrus, green tea, blueberries, bell peppers, and even dark chocolate lend their antioxidant prowess to your defense.

6. Savoring Deep Sleep: Deep sleep is a balm for the weary soul and a tonic for your cellular powerhouses. Cellular repair, ATP production, and hormone regulation unfold during this nocturnal journey, nourishing your mitochondria. ATP (adenosine triphosphate) production refers to the process by which cells generate ATP molecules, which are the primary energy currency of cells. ATP is essential for various cellular activities, including metabolism, muscle contraction, and active transport of molecules across cell membranes.

7. Inviting Movement: Movement becomes a choreography that celebrates mitochondrial health. Cellular engines work with newfound vigor as blood circulation and oxygen delivery improve. The growth of new mitochondria further

fortifies cellular resilience.

9. Basking in Sunlight: Sunlight, the harbinger of life, extends its touch to your mitochondria. Sunlight is a cornerstone of cellular well-being for humans on Earth, by triggering vitamin D production and optimizing circadian rhythms.

10. Grounding: Embrace…the Earth's embrace. You usher in negatively charged electrons through grounding or direct contact with the Earth, nurturing the electron transport chain that powers your cellular engines.

Respiratory Health

Lung health is of paramount importance as our lungs play a crucial role in facilitating the exchange of oxygen and carbon dioxide, supporting our respiratory system, and promoting a general sense of well-being. Maintaining optimal lung health is essential for proper breathing, immune function, and overall physical performance.

Several factors can impact lung health, including environmental pollutants, smoking, respiratory infections, allergies, and sedentary lifestyles. Simply becoming aware, mindful and intentional with ones actions and habits, addressing these factors and adopting healthy habits can significantly improve lung support and enhance respiratory function.

Practices That May Positively Impact Lung Health

1. Avoiding smoking and secondhand smoke: Smoking damages lung tissue and increases the risk of lung-related diseases. Quitting smoking or avoiding exposure to secondhand smoke is crucial for maintaining healthy lungs.

Smoking cannabis or any other herbs can be carcinogenic because the combustion of plant material produces a mixture of chemicals, including carcinogens. Carcinogens are substances that can cause cancer by damaging DNA and other genetic material in cells, leading to the uncontrolled growth of cells that characterize cancer.

When cannabis or herbs are smoked, the smoke contains many of the same harmful chemicals found in tobacco smoke. These include tar, which is a sticky substance that can build up in the lungs and lead to respiratory issues, as well as various carcinogenic compounds such as polycyclic aromatic hydrocarbons (PAHs), benzene, and formaldehyde. When these substances are inhaled, they can damage the cells lining the lungs and other parts of the respiratory system, increasing the risk of developing cancer.

It's important to note that while smoking cannabis or herbs can be harmful to your health, there are alternative methods of consumption, such as cannabis oil and edibles, which do not involve inhaling smoke and can be less harmful. When ingested orally, cannabis oil is metabolized by the liver, where it is converted into a different compound that has a longer-lasting effect compared to smoking or vaporizing cannabis. Oral ingestion of cannabis oil also provides prolonged relief for conditions like chronic pain, epilepsy, and certain neurological disorders. The extended duration of effects is beneficial for individuals like myself who are seeking long-lasting relief without the need for frequent dosing. Cannabis oil can be formulated to contain specific ratios of cannabinoids (like THC and CBD) and terpenes, allowing users to tailor the product to their specific needs. For example, CBD-rich oils are commonly used for medicinal purposes without the psychoactive effects associated with THC.

2. Reducing exposure to pollutants: Minimizing exposure to air pollutants, such as dust, chemicals, and toxins, benefits lung health. Ensuring proper ventilation and using air filters can help reduce indoor air pollution.

3. Regular physical activity: Regular exercise helps improve lung capacity, strengthens respiratory muscles, and enhances overall lung function. Aerobic exercises like brisk walking, jogging, swimming, and cycling can particularly benefit lung health.

4. Practicing deep breathing exercises: Deep breathing exercises, such as diaphragmatic or belly breathing, can strengthen respiratory muscles, increase lung capacity, and promote relaxation. These exercises involve inhaling deeply, allowing

the diaphragm to expand fully, and exhaling slowly.

5. Maintaining good posture: Proper posture supports optimal lung function by allowing the lungs to expand and contract during breathing fully. Sitting and standing upright helps maximize lung capacity and ensures efficient oxygen exchange.

To test lung health and assess respiratory function at home, you can perform the following exercises:

1. Spirometry: Spirometry is a standard lung function test that measures the air you can inhale and exhale forcefully. Portable spirometers are available for home use, allowing you to monitor your lung capacity and track any changes over time.

2. Peak Flow Meter: A peak flow meter measures the maximum speed at which you can exhale air forcefully. It provides a simple way to monitor changes in lung function and detect early signs of breathing difficulties or asthma flare-ups.

3. Breath-holding exercises: Timing how long you can comfortably hold your breath or monitoring how quickly your breathing returns to normal after physical exertion can offer insights into lung health and efficiency.

Here are three different breath-holding exercises:

- *1. Box Breathing:*
  - Sit or lie down comfortably.
  - Inhale deeply through your nose to a count of four.
  - Hold your breath for a count of four.
  - Exhale slowly through your mouth to a count of four.
  - Hold your breath again for a count of four.
  - Repeat the cycle for several rounds, gradually increasing the count if comfortable.

- *2. Progressive Breath Hold:*
  - Sit in a relaxed position.

- Take a deep breath through your nose, filling your lungs.

- Hold your breath for as long as you comfortably can.

- As you continue holding your breath, mentally count the seconds.

- Slowly release your breath through your mouth.

- Rest and recover briefly before repeating the exercise for several rounds.

- *3. High Altitude Simulation:*

  - Find a comfortable position and take a few deep breaths to relax.

  - Take a deep breath in and hold your breath.

  - While holding your breath, gently nod your head up and down or side to side for as long as possible.

  - Once you need to breathe, exhale slowly and take a recovery breath.

  - Rest and recover before attempting another round if desired.

Here's a breath-holding exercise inspired by the Wim Hof Method:

Wim Hof Breath-Hold Technique:

1. Find a comfortable and quiet space to sit or lie down.

2. Take a few deep breaths to relax and center yourself.

3. Inhale deeply through your nose, filling your lungs with as much air as possible.

4. Exhale fully through your mouth, releasing any tension or stress.

5. Without taking another breath, begin a rapid and rhythmic cycle of breaths, inhaling and exhaling through your nose.

6. After about 30-40 quick breaths, take a final deep inhale and let it out naturally.

7. Exhale fully and hold your breath for as long as possible.

8. As you hold your breath, focus on relaxing your body and quieting your mind.

9. Pay attention to any sensations that arise during the breath-hold, but remain calm and present.

10. When you feel the need to breathe again, take a slow and gentle inhale.

11. Exhale and allow your breathing to return to its normal rhythm.

12. Take a moment to rest and observe how you feel after the exercise.

Note: The Wim Hof Method involves additional components such as cold exposure and mindset training. It is only recommended that individuals learn and practice this method under the guidance of a certified instructor for a comprehensive understanding of the technique and its potential effects.

Remember to perform these exercises in a safe and controlled environment and to stop if they make you feel uncomfortable or lightheaded.

Reading Mucus

Reading mucus can provide valuable insights into our respiratory health and overall well-being. Examining mucus, its color, consistency, and accompanying symptoms can offer clues about potential underlying conditions. Here are some general guidelines for interpreting mucus:

1. Color: Clear or white mucus is typically considered normal, indicating a healthy respiratory system. Yellow or green mucus may suggest the presence of an infection, such as a cold or sinusitis. Rusty or brown-colored mucus could be a sign of older blood, while pink or red mucus may indicate fresh blood requiring medical attention.

2. Consistency: Thin and watery mucus is generally associated with normal respiratory function. Thicker and sticky mucus might suggest dehydration or the body's response to an irritant. Excessively thick and sticky mucus could indicate a respiratory infection or chronic condition.

3. Symptoms: Pay attention to any accompanying symptoms, such as coughing, congestion, or fever. These can provide further context for understanding the underlying cause of the mucus.

It's important to note that mucus should be interpreted in conjunction with other symptoms and medical advice. If you have concerns about your mucus or respiratory health, it is always recommended to consult with a healthcare professional for an accurate diagnosis and appropriate treatment.

Digestive Health

Reading and interpreting bowel movements can provide insights into digestive health and well-being. While bowel movements can vary from person to person, there are certain aspects to consider when assessing them:

1. Frequency: Normal bowel movements can range from several times a day to a few times a week. Consistency in your regular pattern is key. Sudden changes in frequency, such as persistent diarrhea or constipation, may indicate an underlying issue that a healthcare professional should evaluate.

2. Form and Texture: Healthy stool is typically well-formed, smooth, and easy to pass. The Bristol Stool Scale is a helpful tool that categorizes stool types from 1 to 7, ranging from hard lumps to watery consistency. Ideally, stools should be within the Type 3 to Type 4 range, resembling a smooth sausage or snake.

3. Color: Normal stool color varies from light to dark brown. Certain foods, medications, or supplements can temporarily influence color. However, persistent abnormal colors like black, red, pale, or clay-colored stools may indicate digestive problems and require medical attention.

4. Odor: Bowel movements usually have a distinct odor due to the breakdown of food in the digestive system. Foul-smelling or unusually strong odors could indicate malabsorption issues, infections, or dietary imbalances.

5. Additional Symptoms: Pay attention to any accompanying symptoms such as abdominal pain, bloating, or changes in appetite. These can provide further context for understanding digestive health.

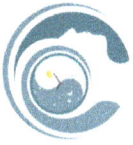

CIRCADIAN360

STOOL CHART

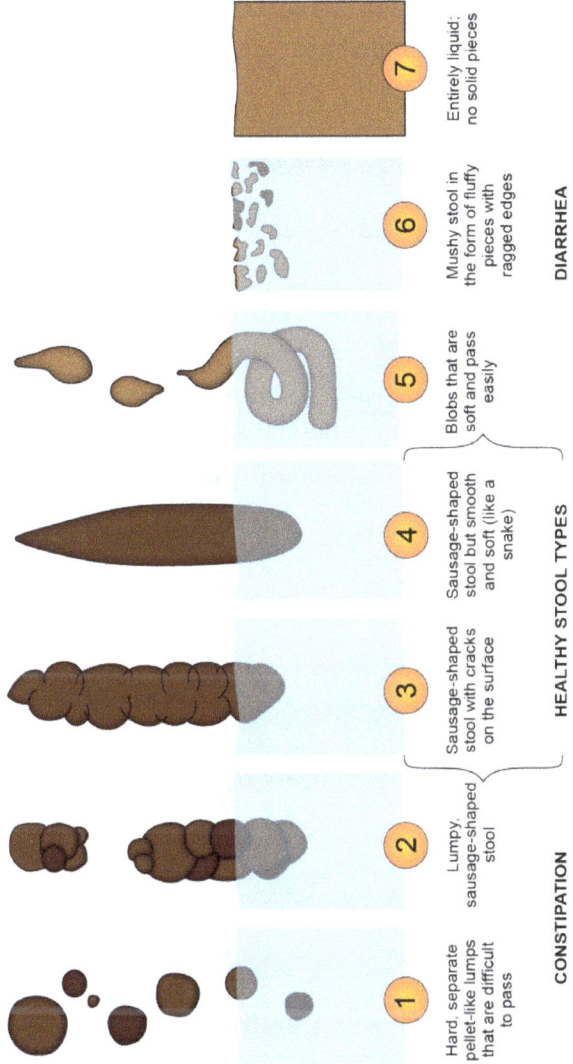

1	2	3	4	5	6	7
Hard separate pellet-like lumps that are difficult to pass	Lumpy, sausage-shaped stool	Sausage-shaped stool with cracks on the surface	Sausage-shaped stool but smooth and soft (like a snake)	Blobs that are soft and pass easily	Mushy stool in the form of fluffy pieces with ragged edges	Entirely liquid; no solid pieces
CONSTIPATION		HEALTHY STOOL TYPES			DIARRHEA	

149

Here is a chart that describes different types of bowel movements and what they can indicate:

Stool Type	Description	Possible Interpretation
Type 1	Separate hard lumps	Constipation, lack of fiber, dehydration
Type 2	Lumpy, sausage-shaped	Mild constipation, inadequate hydration
Type 3	Sausage-shaped with cracks	Normal, healthy bowel movement
Type 4	Sausage-shaped, smooth	Ideal, well-formed stool
Type 5	Soft blobs with clear-cut edges	Lack of fiber, inadequate hydration
Type 6	Fluffy, mushy	Mild diarrhea, dietary intolerance
Type 7	Watery, entirely liquid	Severe diarrhea, digestive disorder, infection

Different bowel colors and what they can potentially indicate:

Stool Color	Possible Interpretation
Brown	Normal, healthy bowel movement

Stool Color	Possible Interpretation
Green	Rapid transit through the digestive system, bile-related issues, or consumption of green-colored foods or dyes
Yellow	Rapid transit, excess fat in the stool, or issues with fat absorption
Black	Upper gastrointestinal bleeding, iron supplements, certain medications, or consumption of black-colored foods
Bright Red	Lower gastrointestinal bleeding, hemorrhoids, anal fissures, or ingestion of red-colored foods
Pale or Clay	Issues with bile flow, liver or gallbladder problems, or certain medications
Grey or White	Lack of bile, liver or gallbladder issues, or problems with fat absorption

These charts are a general guide, and individual experiences may vary. When interpreting bowel movements, it is important to consider other factors such as accompanying symptoms, diet, hydration, and overall health. If you have concerns about your bowel movements or experience persistent digestive issues, consult a healthcare professional for an accurate diagnosis and appropriate treatment.

Drinking With Freshly Squeezed Lemon And Lime Juice In Our Water For Digestive Support

Lemons and limes are citrus fruits rich in vitamin C, citric acid, and other beneficial compounds. When squeezed into water, they can provide a range of potential benefits for the body, including aiding in releasing phlegm and mucus. They work as an astringent, supporting detoxification of the digestive and renal systems, helping to move grease, gas, and bloating, and assisting in liver cleansing. The high vitamin C content in lemons and limes can help to thin and loosen phlegm and mucus, making it easier to expel from the respiratory system. This can be particularly beneficial for those suffering from respiratory conditions such as colds, coughs, and sinus congestion.

Astringent properties: Lemons and limes are natural astringents that can help tighten tissues and reduce inflammation. This can be beneficial for conditions such as sore throats, gum inflammation, and skin issues, as well as helping to tone and cleanse the digestive tract.

Detoxification of digestive and renal systems: The citric acid in lemons and limes can stimulate digestive enzymes, helping to improve digestion and detoxify the digestive system. It can also help to flush out toxins from the renal system, supporting kidney health and function.

Relief from gas, bloating, and grease: The acidic nature of lemons and limes can help to break down fats and promote digestion, which can aid in reducing symptoms of gas, bloating, and indigestion. When mixed with sparkling water, the lemon or lime juice can further help relieve gas and bloating in the digestive system; however, sparkling and/or mineral waters do contribute to increased tartar and tooth calcifications in the mouth. With this, be mindful of maintaining proper, daily oral hygiene, to maintain a consistent habit of brushing away those micro-minerals before they time to build up.

Liver cleansing: Lemons and limes are known to have a cleansing effect on the liver, a vital organ for detoxification. The antioxidants and other beneficial compounds in these citrus fruits can help to support liver function, flush out toxins, and promote liver health.

Individual responses to lemon or lime water may vary. Some people may be sensitive to citrus fruits. So, listening to your body and adjusting it accordingly is essential. Also, consuming lemon or lime water in moderation, as part of a balanced diet, is recommended. Overconsumption of citrus fruits, especially in concentrated forms, can negatively affect tooth enamel and digestive health also...so please, as with all things...practice moderation alongside your proper maintenance practices.

Astringent Fruits And Vegetables

When we zoom out beyond lemons and limes, we discover a category of fruit: **Astringent produce**.

Astringent fruits and vegetables have a puckering or drying effect on the mouth due to their high tannin content. Tannins are naturally occurring compounds found in plants that can bind to proteins and other organic compounds, resulting in a dry and puckering sensation in the mouth. Astringent fruits and vegetables are often described as having a tart, sour, or bitter taste. They are also known to have a drying effect on the tissues with which they come into contact.

Astringent fruits and vegetables can offer several benefits when it comes to detoxing.

Here are some of the potential benefits:

Promote Digestive Health: Astringent fruits and vegetables are rich in compounds such as tannins and flavonoids, which can help to promote digestive health by reducing inflammation and irritation in the gastrointestinal tract.

Improve Skin Health: Astringent fruits and vegetables can also help improve your skin's health. These foods can help to tighten and tone the skin, reducing the appearance of fine lines and wrinkles.

Boost Immunity: Astringent fruits and vegetables are often rich in antioxidants, which can help boost your immune system and protect your body from free radical damage.

Reduce Inflammation: Many astringent fruits and vegetables have anti-inflammatory properties, which can help to reduce inflammation throughout the body.

Aid in Detoxification: Astringent fruits and vegetables can help support your body's natural detoxification processes by promoting the elimination of toxins through the liver and kidneys.

Examples of Astringent Fruits

- Persimmons (Hachiya variety)
- Pomegranates
- Cranberries
- Guava
- Quinces
- Sour cherries
- Green apples
- Blackcurrants
- Lemons
- Limes
- Sloe berries
- Raspberries (unripe)

Examples of Astringent Vegetables

- Artichokes
- Collard greens
- Spinach

- Eggplant (unripe)

- Okra

- Brussels sprouts

- Radicchio

- Beet greens

- Swiss chard

- Endive

Please note that the perception of astringency can vary from person to person. Some fruits or vegetables may be less or more astringent depending on their ripeness and preparation methods. That's why I feel that it's best to always best to try a small amount and see how it suits your taste buds.

Fruits And Vegetables That Are High In Fiber

When it comes to cleansing, the role of fiber-rich fruits and vegetables is primarily to support the body's natural detoxification processes. Fiber helps to move waste products through the digestive system more efficiently and can bind to toxins and promote their excretion from the body; moreover, a diet rich in fruits and vegetables can provide many vitamins, minerals, and antioxidants that support the body's detoxification pathways and overall health.

Fiber-rich foods are beneficial for our health for several reasons:

Digestive health: Fiber helps regulate bowel movements and prevents constipation by adding bulk to stool, promoting regularity, and preventing digestive issues.

Heart health: Diets high in fiber have been associated with a reduced risk of heart disease. In particular, Soluble fiber can help lower LDL (low-density lipoprotein) cholesterol levels, also known as "bad" cholesterol, by binding to cholesterol and promoting its excretion.

Blood sugar management: Fiber can help regulate blood sugar levels by slowing down the absorption of sugar into the bloodstream. This can be particularly beneficial for individuals with diabetes or those at risk of developing diabetes.

Weight management: High-fiber foods are typically low in calories and can help promote satiety or a feeling of fullness, which can help with weight management by reducing overall calorie intake.

Gut microbiota health: Fiber acts as a prebiotic, nourishing beneficial bacteria in our gut, promoting healthy gut microbiota and overall gut health.

Here is a list of fruits, organized from highest fiber count to lowest, along with their fiber content, as well as the vitamins, minerals, and enzymes found in each:

Avocado: Fiber - 10g; Vitamins - Vitamin E, Vitamin K; Minerals - Potassium, Magnesium; Enzymes - Lipase

Raspberry: Fiber - 8g; Vitamins - Vitamin C, Vitamin E; Minerals - Manganese, Folate; Enzymes - N/A

Blackberry: Fiber - 5.3g; Vitamins - Vitamin C, Vitamin K; Minerals - Manganese, Magnesium; Enzymes - N/A

Guava: Fiber - 5.4g; Vitamins - Vitamin C, Vitamin A; Minerals - Manganese, Folate; Enzymes - N/A

Passion fruit: Fiber - 5.4g; Vitamins - Vitamin C, Vitamin A; Minerals - Iron, Magnesium; Enzymes - N/A

Pear: Fiber - 4.3g; Vitamins - Vitamin C, Vitamin K; Minerals - Potassium, Folate; Enzymes - Amylase

Kiwi: Fiber - 3g; Vitamins - Vitamin C, Vitamin K; Minerals - Potassium, Folate; Enzymes - Actinidin

Pomegranate: Fiber - 2.8g; Vitamins - Vitamin C, Vitamin K; Minerals - Folate, Potassium; Enzymes - N/A

Apple: Fiber - 2.4g; Vitamins - Vitamin C, Vitamin K; Minerals - Potassium, Folate; Enzymes - Amylase

Orange: Fiber - 2.3g; Vitamins - Vitamin C, Folate; Minerals - Potassium, Magnesium; Enzymes - N/A

Mango: Fiþer - 1.6g; Vitamins - Vitamin C, Vitamin A; Minerals - Folate, Potassium; Enzymes - N/A

Banana: Fiber - 1.6g; Vitamins - Vitamin C, Vitamin B6; Minerals - Potassium, Magnesium; Enzymes - N/A

Papaya: Fiber - 1.8g; Vitamins - Vitamin C, Vitamin A; Minerals - Folate, Potassium; Enzymes - Papain

Watermelon: Fiber - 0.4g; Vitamins - Vitamin C, Vitamin A; Minerals - Potassium, Magnesium; Enzymes - N/A

Pineapple: Fiber - 0.9g; Vitamins - Vitamin C, Vitamin B6; Minerals - Manganese, Folate; Enzymes - Bromelain

Here is the list of vegetables, organized from highest fiber count to lowest, along with their fiber content, as well as the vitamins, minerals, and enzymes found in each:

Artichoke: Fiber - 10.3g; Vitamins - Vitamin C, Vitamin K; Minerals - Folate, Magnesium; Enzymes - Lipase

Split peas: Fiber - 8.3g; Vitamins - Vitamin B6, Vitamin K; Minerals - Folate, Potassium; Enzymes - Amylase

Lentils: Fiber - 7.9g; Vitamins - Vitamin B6, Vitamin K; Minerals - Folate, Iron; Enzymes - Amylase

Chickpeas: Fiber - 7.6g; Vitamins - Vitamin B6, Vitamin C; Minerals - Folate, Iron; Enzymes - Amylase

Green peas: Fiber - 5g; Vitamins - Vitamin C, Vitamin K; Minerals - Folate,

Iron; Enzymes - Amylase

Okra: Fiber - 3.2g; Vitamins - Vitamin C, Vitamin K; Minerals - Folate, Magnesium; Enzymes - Catalase

Brussels sprouts: Fiber - 3.3g; Vitamins - Vitamin C, Vitamin K; Minerals - Folate, Potassium; Enzymes - Catalase.

Collard greens: Fiber - 4g; Vitamins - Vitamin C, Vitamin K; Minerals - Calcium, Folate; Enzymes - Myrosinase

Eggplant: Fiber - 3g; Vitamins - Vitamin C, Vitamin K; Minerals - Folate, Potassium; Enzymes - N/A

Beetroot: Fiber - 2.8g; Vitamins - Vitamin C, Folate; Minerals - Iron, Potassium; Enzymes - N/A

Broccoli: Fiber - 2.6g; Vitamins - Vitamin C, Vitamin K; Minerals - Folate, Calcium; Enzymes - Myrosinase

Spinach: Fiber - 2.2g; Vitamins - Vitamin A, Vitamin K; Minerals - Folate, Iron; Enzymes - N/A

Carrot: Fiber - 2.1g; Vitamins - Vitamin A, Vitamin K; Minerals - Potassium, Beta-carotene; Enzymes - N/A

Sweet potato: Fiber - 1.8g; Vitamins - Vitamin A, Vitamin C; Minerals - Potassium, Beta-carotene; Enzymes - N/A

Cabbage: Fiber - 1.8g; Vitamins - Vitamin C, Vitamin K; Minerals - Folate, Calcium; Enzymes - Lipase

Green beans: Fiber - 1.8g; Vitamins - Vitamin C, Vitamin K; Minerals - Folate, Potassium; Enzymes - N/A

Asparagus: Fiber - 1.8g; Vitamins - Vitamin C, Vitamin K; Minerals - Folate, Potassium; Enzymes - Asparaginase

Cauliflower: Fiber - 1.9g; Vitamins - Vitamin C, Vitamin K; Minerals - Folate, Calcium; Enzymes - N/A

Turnip: Fiber - 1.8g; Vitamins - Vitamin C, Folate; Minerals - Calcium, Potassium; Enzymes - Lipase

Bell pepper: Fiber - 1.7g; Vitamins - Vitamin C, Vitamin A; Minerals - Folate,

Potassium; Enzymes - N/A

Kale: Fiber - 1.6g; Vitamins - Vitamin C, Vitamin K; Minerals - Folate, Calcium; Enzymes - Myrosinase

Celery: Fiber - 1.6g; Vitamins - Vitamin C, Vitamin K; Minerals - Folate, Potassium; Enzymes - N/A

Radish: Fiber - 1.6g; Vitamins - Vitamin C, Vitamin B6; Minerals - Folate, Potassium; Enzymes - Lipase

Swiss chard: Fiber - 1.6g; Vitamins - Vitamin C, Vitamin K; Minerals - Magnesium, Folate; Enzymes - Myrosinase

Zucchini: Fiber - 1.2g; Vitamins - Vitamin C, Vitamin K; Minerals - Potassium, Magnesium; Enzymes - N/A

Cucumber: Fiber - 0.5g; Vitamins - Vitamin C, Vitamin K; Minerals - Potassium, Magnesium; Enzymes - N/A

Please note that the specific vitamins, minerals, and enzymes may vary in quantity and availability depending on factors such as cooking method, ripeness, and storage conditions of the fruits and vegetables.

Healing Using the Five Sense: Self-Care Routines & Hacks

Healing using the five senses is a powerful and natural way to promote wellness and improve our overall health.

Even small changes in our daily routines can profoundly impact our overall well-being. Incorporating natural and sensory experiences into our daily lives can support our bodies 'natural healing abilities and promote a healthier and more balanced life.

The Tactile System: A Guide to Healing with Touch

Our sense of touch is called the tactile system. It's how we feel all touch sensations, including vibrations, temperature, textures, and pain. We are social creatures, and touch is essential to our social interactions. From a simple handshake to a warm hug, touch is one of the most fundamental ways we communicate and connect; however, many people may experience touch starvation in our modern world, which can profoundly impact our mental and physical health.

Touch starvation occurs when people are deprived of safe, nurturing touch for extended periods. This can be due to various factors, such as living alone, social isolation, or a history of trauma. Touch starvation can lead to anxiety, depression, and even physical illness.

Research has shown that touch can reduce stress, lower blood pressure, and even boost the immune system. When we experience touch, our bodies release hormones such as oxytocin and serotonin, which promote feelings of relaxation and well-being. This is why safe touch therapy is becoming increasingly popular to promote healing.

It must be noted that for some people, touch can be a source of pain and trauma. Childhood experiences with unwanted or abusive touch can have lifelong impacts on our mental health and relationships. For those who have experienced trauma, it's important to seek out therapists and practitioners who specialize in trauma-informed touch therapy. These professionals can help individuals heal from the impacts of early experiences with touch and learn to experience safe, nurturing touch in a comfortable and empowering way.

Safe touch therapy can take many forms. Some examples include massage therapy, reiki, cuddling, and animal-assisted therapy. It's important to find a safe and comfortable therapy and work with a trained and experienced practitioner to provide a safe touch.

In addition to seeking out touch therapy, it's also important to prioritize touch in our daily lives. This can include hugging a loved one, holding hands with a friend, or even patting a pet. We can support our mental and physical health and promote healing by prioritizing safe, nurturing touch.

The Meridian System

Circadian360's
Meridian Body - Anterior & Posterior

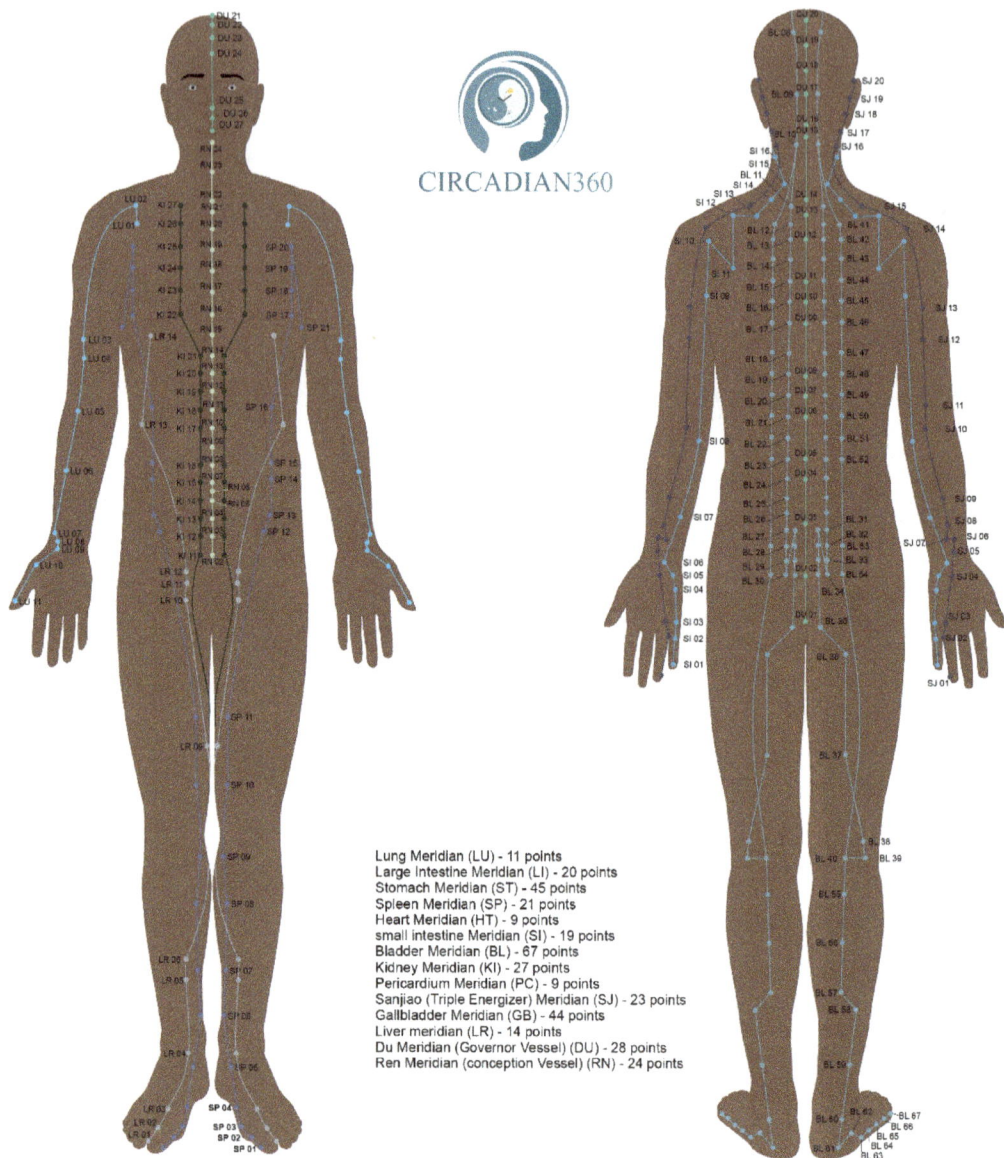

CIRCADIAN360

Lung Meridian (LU) - 11 points
Large Intestine Meridian (LI) - 20 points
Stomach Meridian (ST) - 45 points
Spleen Meridian (SP) - 21 points
Heart Meridian (HT) - 9 points
small intestine Meridian (SI) - 19 points
Bladder Meridian (BL) - 67 points
Kidney Meridian (KI) - 27 points
Pericardium Meridian (PC) - 9 points
Sanjiao (Triple Energizer) Meridian (SJ) - 23 points
Gallbladder Meridian (GB) - 44 points
Liver meridian (LR) - 14 points
Du Meridian (Governor Vessel) (DU) - 28 points
Ren Meridian (conception Vessel) (RN) - 24 points

The meridian system is a concept derived from Traditional Chinese Medicine (TCM) and is believed to be an energy network within the body.

According to TCM, energy, or qi (pronounced "chee"), flows through these meridians, which are pathways that connect various organs and systems. The meridian system is integral to practices like acupuncture, acupressure, and certain forms of tapping therapy.

162

The meridian system is used in TCM to diagnose and treat illnesses. In this system, imbalances or blockages in the flow of qi along the meridians are believed to cause

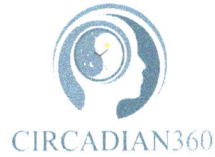

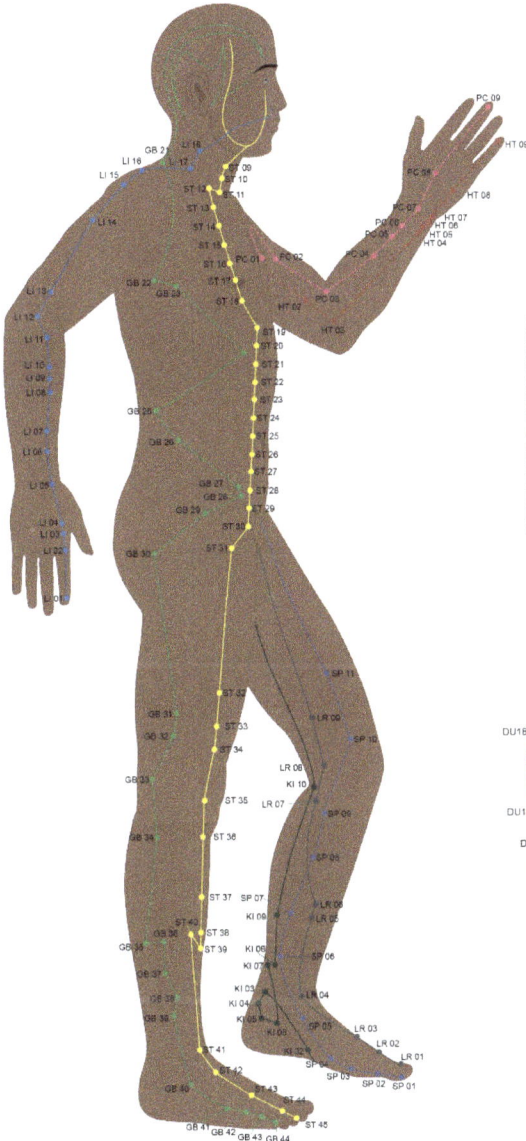

Lung Meridian (LU) - 11 points
Large Intestine Meridian (LI) - 20 points
Stomach Meridian (ST) - 45 points
Spleen Meridian (SP) - 21 points
Heart Meridian (HT) - 9 points
Small Intestine Meridian (SI) - 19 points
Bladder Meridian (BL) - 67 points
Kideny Meridian (KI) - 27 points
Pericardium Meridian (PC) - 9 points
Sanjiao (Tripl Energizer) Meridian (SJ) - 23 points
Gallbladder Meridian (DU) - 44 points
Liver Meridian (LR) - points
Du Meridian (Governor Vessel) (DU) - 28 points
Ren Meridian (Conception Vessel) (RN) - 24 points

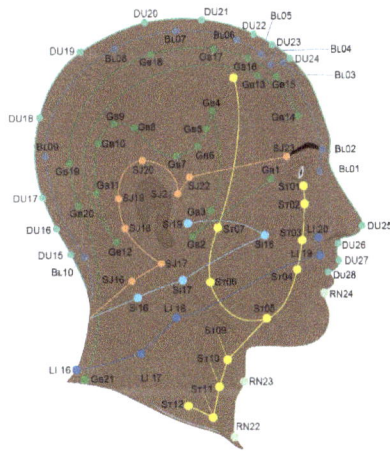

Circadian360's
Meridian Body - Side Body & Head

health issues. By assessing the flow of qi and identifying specific points along the meridians, TCM practitioners can determine patterns of disharmony and develop treatment strategies to restore balance.

Different cultures have their systems of energy pathways, but the meridian system is primarily associated with TCM. While TCM originated in China, it has influenced various East Asian cultures, including Japan and Korea, where similar concepts are used in their respective traditional medical practices.

Observational self-diagnosis/self-assessments using the meridian system involves examining the body and observing sure signs and symptoms that may indicate imbalances in energy flow. Practitioners or individuals familiar with the meridian system may look for physical manifestations such as tenderness or sensitivity at specific acupoints, skin color or texture changes, abnormal sensations, or palpable irregularities along the meridians. These observations can provide clues about potential imbalances or areas of concern within the body.

Including Methods Incorporating The Meridian System, Here Are A Few Different Types Of Touch Therapy

Massage Therapy: Manipulating the body's soft tissues improves circulation, relieves muscle tension and pain, and promotes relaxation.

Acupressure: Applying pressure to specific points on the body to stimulate the body's natural healing abilities and improve overall health.

Reflexology: Applying pressure to specific points on the feet, hands, and ears corresponding to different body parts to relieve pain, reduce stress, and improve overall health.

Reiki: A form of energy healing that involves the laying of hands to balance the body's energy and promote healing.

Craniosacral Therapy: A gentle, hands-on approach that releases tension in the soft tissues surrounding the central nervous system to promote relaxation and improve overall health.

Myofascial Release: A technique that involves applying sustained pressure to the connective tissue to release tension and improve flexibility.

Shiatsu: A form of Japanese massage that involves applying pressure to specific points on the body to relieve tension and improve overall health.

Healing Touch: A form of energy therapy that involves gentle touch to clear and balance the body's energy to promote healing.

Lymphatic Massage: Gentle massage that uses light pressure and rhythmic movements to stimulate the flow of lymphatic fluid throughout the body, helping to remove waste and toxins and boost the immune system. Lymphatic massage is a safe and effective form of touch therapy that can be done by a practitioner or oneself.

Some techniques, such as **dry brushing** and **self-massage**, can be done at home. *Dry brushing* involves using a stiff brush to gently brush the skin toward the lymph nodes, which can help stimulate lymphatic flow. *Self-massage* techniques can involve gentle pressure and circular movements on the neck, armpits, abdomen, and groin areas, where lymph nodes are located. It's important to use gentle pressure and avoid any areas of the body that may be tender or sensitive.

The Importance Of The Lymphatic System & How To Give Yourself A Lymphatic Massage

Circadian360's Lymphatic Body

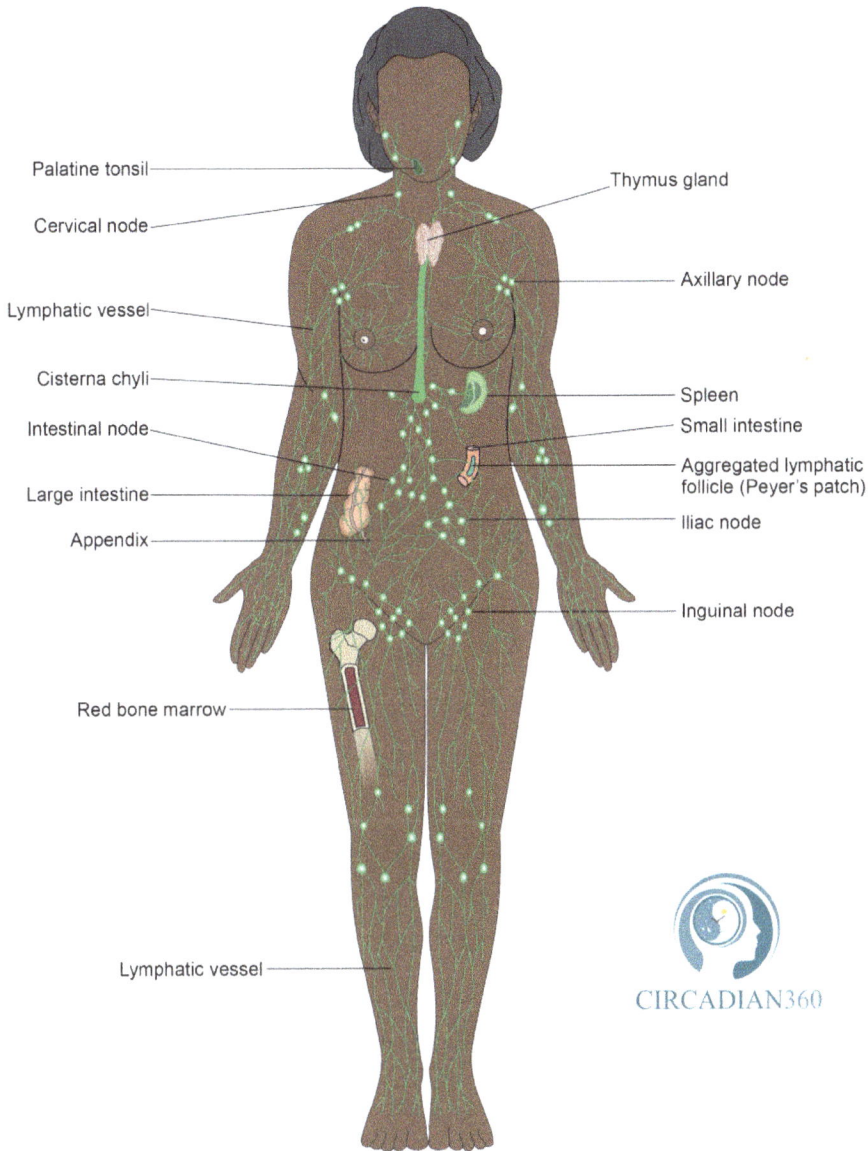

Palatine tonsil

Cervical node

Lymphatic vessel

Cisterna chyli

Intestinal node

Large intestine

Appendix

Red bone marrow

Lymphatic vessel

Thymus gland

Axillary node

Spleen

Small intestine

Aggregated lymphatic follicle (Peyer's patch)

Iliac node

Inguinal node

CIRCADIAN360

The lymphatic system is a network of vessels, nodes, and organs that work together to transport lymph fluid, a clear fluid that contains waste products, toxins, and immune cells throughout the body. The lymphatic system is crucial to immune function and helps remove tissue waste and toxins.

There are several ways to support the health and function of the lymphatic system and encourage lymphatic drainage. Here are some suggestions:

- **Stay hydrated:** Drinking plenty of water helps to keep the lymphatic fluid flowing properly and prevents it from becoming thick and stagnant.

- **Eat a healthy diet:** A diet rich in fruits, vegetables, and whole grains provides essential nutrients that support the lymphatic system. Avoiding processed foods, excessive sugar, and unhealthy fats can help reduce inflammation and support lymphatic function.

- **Exercise regularly:** Physical activity like walking, jogging, or practicing yoga can help stimulate lymphatic flow and promote drainage.

- **Dry brushing:** Using a dry brush with natural bristles, gently brush your skin in circular motions towards the heart before showering. This can help stimulate lymphatic flow and exfoliate the skin.

- **Hot and cold showers:** Alternating between hot and cold water during your shower can help stimulate lymphatic flow. Start with hot water for a few minutes, then switch to cold water for a minute or two. Repeat the process a few times, always ending with cold water.

- **Reduce stress:** Chronic stress can negatively impact the lymphatic system. Stress-reducing activities like meditation, deep breathing, or getting enough restful sleep can help support lymphatic health.

- **Lymphatic massage:** You can perform a gentle self-massage on areas where lymph nodes are concentrated, such as the neck, armpits, and groin. Use light pressure and circular motions towards the heart to help stimulate lymphatic flow.

Here Is A Step-By-Step Guide On How To Give Yourself A Lymphatic Massage:

Step 1: Find a comfortable and quiet space: Choose a space where you can lie down or sit comfortably without distractions.

Step 2: Prepare your body: Ensure your skin is clean and dry. You may choose to use a natural oil, such as coconut or jojoba oil, to help your hands glide smoothly over your skin.

Step 3: Begin at the neck: Start by placing your fingertips on one side of your neck, just below the earlobe. Use *gentle*, circular motions to massage the skin, moving downwards towards the collarbone. Repeat this motion several times, gradually moving towards the center of your neck.

Step 4: Move to the armpits: Place your fingertips in your armpit area and use *gentle* circular motions to massage the skin. The lymph nodes in the armpits are important for draining lymph from the arms and upper body.

Step 5: Massage the chest and breasts: Using light pressure, *gently* massage your chest and breasts in circular motions. Avoid pressing too hard on the breast tissue; always be gentle and mindful of any sensitivity or discomfort.

Step 6: Move to the abdomen: Place your hands on your lower abdomen, just above the pubic bone, and use *gentle*, clockwise circular motions to massage the area. This can help stimulate lymphatic flow in the abdominal area.

Step 7: Massage the limbs: Move to your arms and legs, using long, sweeping motions towards the heart. Start at the fingers and toes and work up, using light pressure and circular motions.

Step 8: Finish with the back: If possible, use a long-handled brush or a foam roller to gently brush or roll along your back, moving from the lower back towards the heart. If you don't have a tool, you can use your hands to massage the skin on your back in circular motions.

Step 9: Drink and rest: After the lymphatic massage, drink plenty of water to help flush out any toxins that may have been mobilized during the massage.

Rest and relax for a while to allow your body to benefit from the massage fully. Always use *gentle* pressure and circular motions during the lymphatic massage, and avoid pressing too hard or causing any pain. If you have any underlying health conditions or concerns, it's best to consult with a healthcare professional before attempting a self-lymphatic massage. They can provide personalized advice and recommendations based on your needs and health status, to make sure your journey is safely and fully supported.

Tapping

Tapping on meridian points as a means of self-care is used in practices like Emotional Freedom Techniques (EFT) and acupuncture. It involves gently tapping on specific points on the body known as meridian points or acupoints. These points are believed to be connected to the body's energy pathways or meridians, as described in Traditional Chinese Medicine (TCM). Tapping on these points while focusing on specific issues or intentions is thought to help restore energy balance and promote overall well-being.

Here are some commonly tapped meridian points, along with their functions and potential benefits:

1. **Hand Tapping Point (Small Intestine Meridian):** This point is located on the side of the hand, between the base of the pinky finger and the wrist. It is often used as the setup point in tapping. It is believed to help release negative emotions and improve self-acceptance.

2. **Top of the Head (Governing Vessel Meridian):** This point is located on the crown of the head. Tapping on this point promotes clarity, focus, and a sense of empowerment.

3. **Eyebrow (Bladder Meridian):** The point is located at the beginning of the eyebrow, near the bridge of the nose. Tapping here may help relieve tension, promote mental clarity, and release negative thoughts or beliefs.

4. **Side of the Eye (Gallbladder Meridian):** This point is on the bone at the outer corner of the eye. Tapping here supports decision-making, reduces fear, and releases emotional stress.

5. **Under the Eye (Stomach Meridian):** This point is located on the bone just

below the center of the eye. Tapping on this point may help alleviate anxiety, worry, and digestive issues.

6. **Under the Nose (Governing Vessel Meridian):** This point is between the nose and upper lip. Tapping here is thought to reduce stress, promote relaxation, and increase self-acceptance.

7. **Chin Point (Central Vessel Meridian):** This point is between the lower lip and the chin. Tapping on this point may help release emotional blockages, promote emotional stability, and relieve feelings of guilt or shame.

8. **Collarbone (Kidney Meridian):** This point is just below the collarbone, where it meets the breastbone. Tapping here may help balance energy, reduce anxiety, and improve emotional stability.

9. **Under the Arm (Spleen Meridian):** This point is on the side of the body, about four inches below the armpit. Tapping here may help reduce stress, boost energy, and enhance emotional well-being.

10. **Inside of the Wrist (Pericardium Meridian):** This point is on the inner side of the wrist, in line with the little finger. Tapping here promotes emotional balance, relieves stress, and supports heart health.

When tapping on these meridian points, repeating affirmations, statements, or reminders related to the specific issue or intention you are addressing is common. The combination of tapping and focused attention on the issue is thought to help release emotional and energetic blockages, reduce stress, and promote a sense of calm and well-being.

It's important to note that tapping on meridian points can be a valuable self-care practice for some individuals. It may not work the same way for everyone.

Trigger Point Therapy

Trigger point therapy, also known as myofascial trigger point therapy, focuses on identifying and releasing trigger points in the muscles. Trigger points are hypersensitive areas within muscle fibers that can cause pain and discomfort, often referring to pain in other body parts. During trigger point therapy, pressure is applied to these points to release tension and alleviate pain.

While trigger point therapy and tapping involve physical contact with the body, they target different objectives. Trigger point therapy primarily addresses muscular tension and pain, while tapping techniques are more commonly used for emotional and psychological well-being. I was introduced to trigger point therapy when I had muscle knots, and I began using various foam rollers and devices traditionally reserved for athletic performance and recovery. In these efforts, I was able to release tension, toxins and knotted muscle strains, eventually finding relief.

In acupuncture and acupressure, these trigger points are often aligned with the meridian system, a network of energy pathways believed to circulate through the body. These meridians are associated with different organs and systems, and acupoints along these meridians are believed to have specific effects when stimulated.

Foot Soak

Foot soaking is a practice that involves immersing the feet in a tub of water mixed with various ingredients, such as salts, herbs, and other beneficial substances. It is known to have several benefits for physical health, relaxation, and spiritual well-being. Throughout history, many cultures have used foot soaking as a spiritual practice to cleanse, purify, and heal the body and mind.

Many Cultures Worldwide Have Used Foot Soaking As A Spiritual Practice For Centuries.

For example:

Ancient Chinese Medicine: In Traditional Chinese Medicine, foot soaking is considered a form of hydrotherapy and is believed to help balance the body's energy, or qi, and improve overall health and well-being.

Native American traditions: Some Native American tribes use foot soaking as a purification ritual in sweat lodge ceremonies to cleanse the body and mind and promote spiritual healing.

Ayurveda: In Ayurvedic medicine, a traditional system from India, foot soaking with specific herbs or oils is believed to help balance the doshas (energetic forces) in the body and promote overall health and vitality.

Benefits of foot soaking

Relaxation and stress relief: Foot soaking can help relax the muscles and joints in the feet, reducing tension and stress. It can also promote overall relaxation and a sense of well-being, which can be beneficial for managing stress and anxiety.

Improved circulation: Warm foot soaks can promote blood flow to the feet, which can improve circulation and relieve cold feet, numbness, and swelling. This can particularly benefit individuals with poor circulation or certain medical conditions, such as diabetes.

Detoxification: Foot soaking with certain ingredients, such as Epsom salt, can help draw out toxins from the body through the feet, helping to detoxify the body and promote a sense of purification and renewal.

Softening and exfoliation of the skin: Foot soaking can help soften the skin of the feet, making it easier to exfoliate and remove dead skin cells. This can result in smoother, healthier-looking feet.

Relief from foot ailments: Foot soaking with specific ingredients, such as herbs or essential oils, can help alleviate foot ailments such as foot fungus, foot odor, and soreness and promote overall foot health.

Different foot soaks can be prepared using various ingredients, including salts, herbs, and other beneficial substances.

Here are some examples:

Epsom salt foot soak: Epsom salt, a form of magnesium sulfate, is known for its muscle-relaxing properties. It can help relieve soreness and tiredness in the feet. To prepare an Epsom salt foot soak, dissolve half a cup of Epsom salt in warm water and soak your feet for about 15-20 minutes.

Magnesium salt foot soak: Magnesium salt, also known as magnesium chloride, is another type of salt that can be used for foot soaking. It is believed to help promote relaxation, reduce inflammation, and improve overall foot health. Dissolve half a cup of magnesium salt in warm water and soak your feet for 15-20 minutes.

Herbal foot soak: Herbs such as chamomile, lavender, rosemary, and peppermint can be used to prepare a relaxing and soothing herbal foot soak. You can use fresh or dried herbs and steep them in warm water for about 10 minutes before soaking your feet. You can also use a muslin bag or a foot soak basin with a built-in herb compartment for easy clean-up.

Antifungal foot soak: Foot soaking with antifungal herbs such as tea tree oil, oregano oil, or thyme can help combat foot fungus and promote foot health. Add a few drops of these essential oils to a tub of warm water and a handful of Epsom salt, and soak your feet for about 15-20 minutes to create an antifungal foot soak.

Oatmeal foot soak: Oatmeal is known for its soothing and moisturizing properties, making it an excellent ingredient for a foot soak. Grind half a cup of oatmeal into a fine powder and add it to warm water. Soak your feet for 15-20 minutes to help soothe dry, irritated skin and promote overall foot health.

Here are 5-foot soak recipes that combine salts, herbs, and other beneficial ingredients:

Relaxing Lavender Foot Soak:

1/2 cup Epsom salt

1/4 cup dried lavender flowers

5-10 drops of lavender essential oil

Dissolve Epsom salt in warm water, and add dried lavender flowers and lavender essential oil. Soak your feet for 15-20 minutes for a relaxing and calming experience.

Invigorating Peppermint Foot Soak:

1/2 cup magnesium salt

1/4 cup fresh or dried peppermint leaves

5-10 drops of peppermint essential oil

Dissolve magnesium salt in warm water, add peppermint leaves and essential oil. Soak your feet for 15-20 minutes for a refreshing and invigorating foot soak.

Detoxifying Tea Tree Oil Foot Soak:

1/2 cup Epsom salt

5-10 drops tea tree essential oil

One tablespoon of apple cider vinegar

Dissolve Epsom salt in warm water, and add tea tree essential oil and apple cider vinegar. Soak your feet for 15-20 minutes to help detoxify and purify your feet.

Soothing Chamomile and Calendula Foot Soak:

1/2 cup oatmeal

1/4 cup dried chamomile flowers

1/4 cup dried calendula flowers

Add dried chamomile and calendula flowers to grind oatmeal into a fine powder. Steep in warm water for 10 minutes, then soak your feet for 15-20 minutes to soothe and moisturize dry, irritated skin.

Revitalizing Rosemary and Lemon Foot Soak:

1/2 cup Epsom salt

Two sprigs of fresh rosemary

Zest of 1 lemon

Dissolve Epsom salt in warm water, and add fresh rosemary sprigs and lemon zest. Soak your feet for 15-20 minutes to refresh and revitalize tired feet.

Note: Before using any foot soak, check for any allergies or sensitivities to the ingredients, and consult with a healthcare professional if you have any underlying health conditions or concerns. Be mindful of any open sores, ulcers, wounds, scars, scrapes and/or scratches that may become irritated when in contact with your foot soak ingredients.

Dry Brushing

Dry brushing is a self-care practice that involves using a dry, stiff-bristled brush to gently brush the skin, typically in a specific pattern, without using water or any other product. The brushing motion is typically directed towards the heart, starting from the extremities and moving towards the body's core.

There are several potential self-care benefits associated with dry brushing, including:

Exfoliation: Dry brushing can help to exfoliate the skin by removing dead skin cells, which can leave the skin looking fresher and smoother.

Improved circulation: The brushing motion of dry brushing can help to stimulate blood circulation, which may help to bring more oxygen and nutrients to the skin and promote a healthy, glowing complexion.

Lymphatic support: Proponents of dry brushing claim that it can help support lymphatic health by stimulating the lymphatic system, which filters waste and toxins from the body; however, more scientific research is needed to fully understand the extent of the impact of dry brushing on the lymphatic system.

Relaxation: Dry brushing can be a relaxing self-care practice that may help reduce stress and promote well-being.

Smoothed skin: Regular dry brushing may help to reduce the appearance of rough, dry skin and ingrown hairs, leaving the skin feeling softer and smoother.

The Olfactory System: A Guide to Healing with the Nose

The olfactory sense is the ability to detect and perceive different odors or smells using the nose. Aromatherapy is a holistic approach to healing that has been used for centuries to improve emotional and physical well-being. It involves using essential oils, handcrafted incense, and other aromatic herbs to promote relaxation, reduce stress, and improve mood. The sense of smell is closely linked to our memories and emotions, which is why aromatherapy can be such a powerful tool for healing.

Essential Oils

Essential oils are extracted from plants and are highly concentrated. They are used in aromatherapy to enhance the effects of massage, baths, and other relaxation techniques. Essential oils can be traced back to ancient Egypt, where they were used for medicinal and cosmetic purposes. Today, essential oils are widely used in aromatherapy to treat various health issues, from anxiety and depression to insomnia and pain.

Perfumes, colognes, and fragrances possess a science beyond mere scents. These aromatic compounds can carry positive or negative energies, adding an intriguing dimension to their effects. High-quality essential oils, renowned for their therapeutic grade, stand out among natural substances due to their remarkable vibrational frequencies ranging from 52 to 320 MHz. Their potential to transform surroundings into hostile environments for disease-causing agents is extraordinary, a feat attributed to their elevated frequencies.

The key is found within selecting top-notch essential oils, as the vibrational levels significantly impact personal frequencies. Lower-grade oils can introduce negativity and even cause allergies. Despite their relatively higher cost, prioritizing therapeutic grade options ensures longevity and optimal benefits with just a few drops.

Inhaling essential oils creates captivating effects by engaging the brain's olfactory nerve cells and the limbic system, which is responsible for emotions, memory, and stimulation. Heightened alertness or deep relaxation can be experienced depending on the chosen oil. These oils offer emotional relief, dissolve negative memories, and enhance cognitive function. They even combat stress effectively, making them essential tools for overcoming life's challenges.

When applied topically, essential oils become potent antioxidants that counteract oxidative damage caused by free radicals. The body absorbs their antioxidant properties upon skin application, improving immunity, mood elevation, and revitalized energy. This application method unveils a revitalizing elixir for holistic well-being.

Essential oils extend benefits beyond the physical realm. They cleanse cell-surface receptors and even possess the potential to reprogram DNA and RNA. Some, like cinnamon, clove, and oregano oils, effectively combat pathogens and microbes. These oils aid the body's natural healing and restorative mechanisms, relieving depression, mood disorders, and dementia. They bring about both relaxation and alertness, contributing to overall happiness.

Distinguishing exceptional essential oils by vibrational frequency, Bruce Tainio's research found rose oil to reign with an astonishing 320 MHz. Helichrysum and lavender followed with 181 MHz and 118 MHz, respectively.

Other essential oils and their frequencies include:

- Peppermint Essential Oil: 78 MHz

- Myrrh Essential Oil: 105 MHz

- Lavender Essential Oil: 118 MHz

- Frankincense Essential Oil: 147 MHz

- Rose Essential Oil: 320 MHz

Highlighted in more depth, rose essential oil's rarity and high frequency of 320 MHz make it a sought-after elixir. It enhances skin health, promotes hormonal balance, and even aids depression and anxiety disorders through aromatherapy. With its 181 MHz frequency, Helichrysum essential oil shines in antibacterial, anti-inflammatory, and wound-healing properties. It supports heart, lung, and overall health, and some attribute potential cancer prevention to it. At 118 MHz, lavender essential oil soothes, relaxes, and aids sleep while benefiting diabetes prevention and brain health.

The exceptional power of essential oils, encompassing their vibrational frequencies and interactions with emotions and thoughts, offers a pathway to profound well-being and vitality. Through conscious choices and practices, elevating personal energy becomes achievable, leading to a more vibrant and fulfilling life.

Ancient Practice of Handcrafted Incense

Like aromatherapy, the ancient practice of hand-making incense involves carefully selecting and blending natural aromatic ingredients to create fragrant compositions. It is an art form passed down through generations in various cultures and is still practiced today. Handmade incense is often revered for its therapeutic and healing properties, mainly through the sense of smell, known as the olfactory sense.

Hand-making incense typically involves gathering or sourcing high-quality raw materials such as resins, herbs, spices, flowers, and woods. These ingredients are carefully chosen for their unique scents and potential therapeutic benefits. The selected ingredients are ground or finely chopped to create a consistent texture.

Next, a binding agent or combustible base material, such as makko (a natural tree bark powder), is added to hold the mixture together. The aromatic ingredients are then blended with the base material, often using traditional techniques like hand mixing or grinding in a mortar and pestle. This blending process requires precision and a deep understanding of the desired scent profiles and therapeutic effects.

Once the mixture is well-blended, it can be shaped into cones, sticks, coils, or pellets, depending on the desired form of incense. The handmade incense is left to dry and cure, allowing the ingredients to harmonize and mature, enhancing their aromatic qualities.

When the handmade incense is burned, it releases fragrant smoke that carries the therapeutic scents into the surrounding environment. As the smoke is inhaled, the olfactory receptors in the nose detect the aromatic molecules, sending signals to the brain's limbic system, which is responsible for emotions, memories, and physiological responses. This direct connection between the olfactory sense and the limbic system is why scents can profoundly affect our emotions, mood, and overall well-being.

Different aromatic ingredients have been traditionally associated with specific healing properties. For example, lavender is often used for relaxation and stress relief, while sandalwood is believed to promote mental clarity and spiritual connection. Frankincense and myrrh have been used for their purifying and grounding effects. Each ingredient brings a unique scent and therapeutic qualities, creating a synergistic blend supporting healing and well-being.

The use of handmade incense in healing practices extends beyond the olfactory sense. The ritual of burning incense can create a sacred and meditative ambiance, fostering a sense of calm, focus, and spiritual connection. The visual element of watching the smoke rise and dissipate can also enhance the overall sensory experience.

The Visual System: A Guide to Healing Using Color Therapy

Color therapy, also known as chromotherapy, is a holistic approach to healing that uses different colors to restore balance and promote physical and emotional well-being. Colors are a form of energy that can affect our moods, emotions, and even our physical health. By incorporating color therapy into our daily lives, we can harness the power of color to support our overall health and well-being.

Each color has its unique energy and can be used to address different physical and emotional concerns. For example, blue is often associated with calmness and relaxation, while red is associated with energy and stimulation. Green is associated with balance and harmony, while yellow is associated with mental clarity and focus. By understanding the properties of different colors, we can use them to create a healing environment that supports our specific needs.

One of the key benefits of color therapy is its ability to balance the energy centers in our body, also known as chakras.

Each chakra is associated with a specific color. By using that color in our environment, we can help to balance and heal that chakra. For example, the heart chakra is associated with the color green. So, surrounding ourselves with green objects or clothing can help balance and heal the heart chakra.

Incorporating color therapy into our daily lives can be as simple as adding a few colorful objects to our environment or clothing in specific colors. For a more targeted approach, color therapy can also be used with other healing modalities, such as massage or acupuncture, to promote more profound healing.

There are many ways to incorporate color therapy into our lives. One of the simplest and most effective is through the use of color visualization. By visualizing different colors, we can tap into their healing properties and promote a sense of calm and well-being. For example, if we are anxious, we can visualize the color blue, associated with calmness and relaxation. By visualizing blue and surrounding ourselves with blue objects, we can help promote a sense of calm and reduce anxiety.

In addition to visualization, there are many other ways to incorporate color therapy into our daily lives. This includes using colored light bulbs in our home or office, wearing clothing in specific colors, or even painting our walls in different colors to create a healing environment. Essential oils can also be used in conjunction with color therapy, as different oils are associated with different colors and can help to enhance the healing properties of those colors.

Color therapy can be a powerful tool for healing. It also can be easily incorporated into our daily lives. Understanding the properties of different colors and using them to create a healing environment can promote physical and emotional well-being and restore balance.

Here is a chart that lists colors and their commonly associated benefits:

Color	Benefits
Red	Red increases energy, passion, and excitement. It can also stimulate the appetite and promote action. Red light therapy, also known as low-level laser therapy (LLLT) or photobiomodulation (PBM), is a therapeutic technique that uses red or near-infrared light to stimulate, heal, and regenerate body tissues. This form of therapy has been studied and used for various purposes, including wound healing, pain relief, reducing inflammation, improving skin conditions, and promoting overall wellness.
Orange	Orange promotes creativity, joy, and enthusiasm. It can also increase energy and appetite.
Yellow	Yellow boosts mood, self-esteem, and confidence. It can also improve concentration and mental clarity.
Green	Green promotes balance, harmony, and growth. It can also have a calming effect on the nervous system.
Blue	Blue induces relaxation, peace, and tranquility. It can also promote communication and self-expression.
Purple	Purple enhances spiritual awareness, intuition, and creativity. It can also promote emotional balance and relaxation.
Pink	Pink encourages feelings of love, warmth, and nurturing. It can also promote feelings of peace and calmness.

Color	Benefits
White	White is associated with clarity. It can also promote feelings of peace and balance.
Black	Black represents power, sophistication, and elegance. It can also promote grounding and emotional protection.

It's important to note that individual perceptions and experiences with color can vary, and cultural and personal associations with colors may also affect their effects. This chart is simply providing a general guide to commonly associated benefits; nevertheless, trusting your intuition and experiences with color is always important.

Here is a chart that lists sound frequencies, chakras, and body systems associated with each color. The chart is based on the principles of various traditional systems of medicine, including Ayurveda, Traditional Chinese Medicine (TCM), and the chakra system from Indian and yogic traditions. The specific associations between colors, chakras, and body systems have been developed through centuries of observation and practice in these traditional systems of medicine.:

Color	Sound Frequency	Chakra	Body System
Red	396 Hz	Root	Adrenal glands, kidneys, and spinal column
Orange	417 Hz	Sacral	Reproductive system, bladder, and lower back

Color	Sound Frequency	Chakra	Body System
Yellow	528 Hz	Solar Plexus	The digestive system, liver, and pancreas
Green	639 Hz	Heart	The circulatory system and lungs
Blue	741 Hz	Throat	Respiratory system and thyroid gland
Indigo	852 Hz	Third Eye	Brain and nervous system
Violet	963 Hz	Crown	The pituitary gland and cerebral cortex

Each color can be used to balance and align the corresponding chakra and body system. For example, listening to 639 Hz or surrounding yourself with green colors can help balance the heart chakra and support the circulatory system and lungs.

It's important to note that color therapy and sound therapy should not replace medical treatment but should be considered as complementary wellness support.

The Auditory System: A Guide to Healing Using Sound

Our environment can profoundly impact our health and well-being, both physically and mentally. Positive environments and people can benefit our health, while negative environments and people can lead to negative outcomes. Unfortunately, many of us are born and raised in unbalanced environments, and we may not even realize it until we step outside on our home settings. In some cases, people may not have experienced what it is like to be in a genuinely positive, immersive environment, making it difficult to know how to fix their health.

Have you ever noticed how the sounds and vibrations around you affect your mood and energy levels? Whether we realize it or not, the vibration and frequency of our environments profoundly impact our well-being. Negative people and environments can drain our energy, while the sounds of nature and positive environments can be incredibly healing. Studies have shown that being in nature and participating in gardening can reduce stress and improve mood.

Instead of using headphones to listen to our favorite songs to escape from negative environments, we can listen to certain frequencies that have been shown to impact our health positively. By incorporating sound therapy into our daily lives, we can reset our body's natural rhythms and start feeling mentally and physically better. With the power of sound therapy, we can take the first step towards a healthier, more balanced life.

Sound healing has been used for thousands of years in cultures worldwide to influence the environments around them. From the chanting of Tibetan monks to the use of singing bowls, sound has been recognized for its therapeutic properties. Sound therapy is still used to promote relaxation, reduce stress and anxiety, and improve overall well-being.

So, how does sound healing work? As Circadian360 has detailed, everything in the universe comprises vibration and frequency, including our bodies. Vibrations and frequencies can help balance and align our bodies' natural energy systems when exposed to certain frequencies. This is where binaural beats come in. Binaural beats are created when two different frequencies are played in each ear, causing the brain to perceive a third, "phantom" frequency. This third frequency can have different effects on the body, depending on its frequency.

Here is a list of frequencies and their potential benefits:

Sound Frequency	Potential Benefits
174 Hz	• It reduces and relieves body pain, stress, and tension.
285 Hz	• It is said to improve energy and motivation.
396 Hz	• It is associated with reducing feelings of guilt and fear.
417 Hz	• Support transitions, righting wrongs, releasing traumas, and stagnant negativity.
432 Hz	• The Sound of the Universe! This is said to be the frequency of the universe or the Miracle Frequency, promoting balance, harmony, and creativity in the mind and body.
528 Hz	• The Love Frequency promotes healing, DNA repair, mental clarity, peace, and joy.
639 Hz	• The Connection Frequency helps improve communication, relationships, and understanding, creating peace and harmony. Ideal also for rekindling and reconnecting.
741 Hz	• The Awakening Frequency aids detoxification, boosts the immune system, and promotes overall well-being. It is also called awakening because we may have "ah ha" moments with this frequency, helping us find solutions to difficult situations.
852 Hz	• The Intuition Frequency aids in improving intuition and promoting spiritual growth.

Sound Frequency	Potential Benefits
963 Hz	Pineal Gland Activation: It is often suggested that the 963Hz frequency can help activate the pineal gland, sometimes called the "third eye." This is thought to enhance intuition, spiritual awareness, and a deeper connection to one's higher self. Higher Consciousness: Advocates claim that listening to or meditating with the 963Hz frequency can facilitate a shift to a higher state of consciousness, promoting feelings of unity, oneness, and a connection to the universe. Emotional Healing: It is believed that exposure to the 963Hz frequency can help release negative emotions, stress, and tension, leading to emotional healing and a sense of tranquility. DNA Repair: Some proponents assert that the 963Hz frequency can support DNA repair and cellular healing, potentially leading to improved physical health. Energetic Balance: The frequency is also thought to balance and align the body's energy centers (chakras), promoting overall harmony and well-being.

While certain frequencies and vibrations can benefit our health, some can be harmful and negatively affect our bodies.

Many popular music genres, such as rock, pop, and even hip-hop, are often unknowingly produced with specific frequencies that can cause disturbances in our bodies and minds. For example, some of these frequencies may be associated with anxiety, stress, or depression.

One of the most discussed frequencies in recent years is 5G, a type of wireless technology that uses high-frequency radio waves to transmit data.

While some argue that it is harmless, many researchers have expressed concern about the potential risks associated with 5G exposure, including increased cancer risk, neurological damage, and reproductive harm. Today, increased mounting concerns about other harmful frequencies, such as those emitted by cell towers, Wi-Fi routers, and microwaves, have been linked to various negative health effects.

Studies have shown that exposure to these harmful frequencies can cause disruptions on a cellular level, leading to oxidative stress, DNA damage, and inflammation, among other issues. Prolonged exposure to these harmful frequencies can also cause sleep disturbances, headaches, fatigue, and other symptoms.

It's important to note that while it may be difficult to avoid exposure to these frequencies in our modern world, taking steps to minimize exposure, such as turning off electronics when not in use and avoiding proximity to cell towers and other radiation sources, can be beneficial.

Whether you choose to listen to binaural beats or other forms of sound therapy, it's clear that the vibrations and frequencies of sound have a powerful effect on our bodies and minds.

The next time you're feeling stressed or need a pick-me-up, try immersing yourself in the healing sounds of nature or explore the world of sound therapy. Your body and mind will thank you.

The Gustatory System: A Guide to Healing Using Taste

Food is integral to our lives, providing sustenance, nourishment, and pleasure. What we eat not only affects our physical health but also our emotional well-being. Our sense of taste is one of the most powerful tools to guide us toward foods that will help us thrive. Understanding the different tastes and flavors can help us make informed choices about what we put in our bodies, leading to a healthier and happier life.

The Six Tastes in Traditional Medicine

Traditional systems of medicine, such as Ayurveda and Traditional Chinese Medicine (TCM), have long recognized the importance of taste in maintaining optimal health. According to Ayurveda, there are six primary tastes: sweet, sour, salty, pungent, bitter, and astringent. Each taste has unique properties and can impact the body differently. Similarly, TCM recognizes five tastes: sweet, sour, bitter, salty, and umami.

Sweet: The sweet taste is associated with earth and water elements. It is said to be nourishing and grounding. In Ayurveda, the sweet taste is believed to strengthen the body and promote longevity. Excessive consumption of sweet foods can lead to imbalances such as weight gain, diabetes, and lethargy.

Sour: The sour taste is associated with fire and is believed to stimulate digestion and increase appetite. In TCM, the sour taste is associated with the liver and can help detoxify the body. Excessive consumption of sour foods can lead to imbalances such as acid reflux and heartburn.

Salty: The salty taste is associated with water and is believed to promote hydration and electrolyte balance. In TCM, the salty taste is associated with the kidneys and can help regulate blood pressure. Excessive consumption of salty foods can lead to imbalances such as high blood pressure and fluid retention.

Pungent: The pungent taste is associated with air and is believed to stimulate metabolism and circulation. In Ayurveda, the pungent taste is believed to promote sweating and detoxification. Excessive consumption of pungent foods can lead to imbalances such as excessive thirst and sweating.

Bitter: The bitter taste is associated with ether and air. It is believed to have a cooling and drying effect on the body. In Ayurveda, the bitter taste is believed to detoxify and purify the body. Excessive consumption of bitter foods can lead to imbalances such as anemia and malnutrition.

Astringent: The astringent taste is associated with air and earth. It is believed to have a binding and drying effect on the body. In Ayurveda, the astringent taste promotes healing and can be used to stop bleeding and diarrhea. Excessive consumption of astringent foods can lead to imbalances such as constipation and dryness.

In addition to Ayurveda and TCM, many other cultures have developed systems of herbalism and nutrition based on their understanding of taste and health. Traditional Native American medicine emphasizes the importance of balance in all aspects of life, including diet. Traditional African medicine uses herbs and plants to treat various health conditions, including diabetes, hypertension, and digestive disorders.

Modern Science and Taste

Recent research has shown that the six tastes recognized in Ayurveda and the five in TCM have a basis in modern science.

Studies have shown that the bitter taste is associated with phytonutrients that have anti-inflammatory and antioxidant properties. The umami taste is associated with glutamate, an amino acid important for brain function, and has been shown to improve cognitive function in elderly individuals. The sweet taste has been associated with the release of serotonin, a neurotransmitter that plays a role in mood regulation.

Modern science has also revealed the importance of the gut microbiome concerning taste and overall health. The microbes in our gut play a crucial role in the metabolism and breakdown of nutrients, including taste-related ones. Studies have shown that the composition of our gut microbiome can impact our taste preferences and even influence our food choices.

The connection between taste and health is a complex and fascinating topic across multiple cultures and disciplines. By understanding the role of taste in different systems of medicine and modern science, we can make informed choices about our diet and optimize our overall health and well-being.

CIRCADIAN360

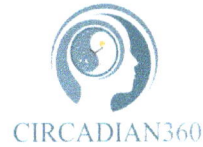

Circadian360's
Tongue Health Guide

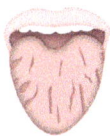

FISSURES
Tongue fissures are a common symptom in 6% to 20% of patients with psoriasis skin disorder.

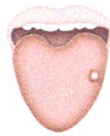

PAINLESS BUMP (S)
A painless bump that appears on the side of the tongue & goes away in 2 weeks or less is not a cause for alarm; however, if it persists longer, it could be an early sign of oral cancer.

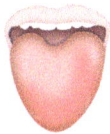

ABNORMAL SMOOTHNESS
Abnormal Smoothness of the tongue is known as atrophic glossitis (AG).

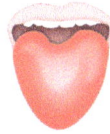

BRIGHT REDNESS
A bright red tongue could be a symptom of a vitamin B12 deficiency.

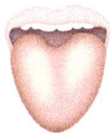

THICK YELLOW COATING
A thick yellow coating on the tongue might be indicative of excess bacterial activity.

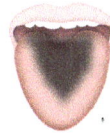

BLACK AND HAIRY
A black and hairy tongue might be caused by excessive smoking and poor oral hygiene.

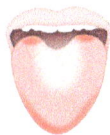

WHITE CREAMY LAYER/PATCHES
A white, cottage cheese-like coating on the tongue is one of the most common symptoms of "oral candidiasis" (OC)-a yeast infection of the mouth.

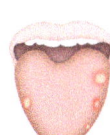

SORES
Tongue sores usually result from eating something sharp or from accidentally biting your tongue; however, they may also signal stress, anxiety or a hormonal imbalance.

For centuries, tongue diagnosis and teeth charting have been used in Traditional Chinese Medicine (TCM) and other alternative healing systems.

Tongue diagnosis examines the tongue's color, shape, coating, and other characteristics to gain insights into a person's overall health. In TCM, the tongue is believed to reflect the condition of the internal organs and provide information about the body's energetic balance. For example, a thick coating on the tongue may indicate an excess of dampness or phlegm in the body, while a pale tongue may suggest a deficiency of qi or blood. TCM practitioners commonly use tongue diagnosis in their diagnostic process and treatment planning.

Tongue diagnosis is a subjective assessment and interpretation of the tongue's color, shape, coating, and other characteristics, according to Traditional Chinese Medicine (TCM) principles.

A step-by-step guide on how to assess the tongue based on tongue appearance

Step 1: Observe the tongue's color

- Look at the tongue's overall color. In TCM, the tongue's color is believed to reflect the condition of the body's internal organs.

- A normal tongue is typically pale pink with a thin, white coating.

- A red tongue may indicate heat or inflammation in the body.

- A pale or bluish tongue may suggest a deficiency of qi or blood.

Step 2: Examine the tongue's coating

- If present, note the thickness, color, and distribution of the tongue's coating.

- A thin, white coating is considered normal in TCM.

- A thick, yellow coating may suggest excess heat or dampness in the body.

- A thick, white coating may indicate a cold or deficient condition.

Step 3: Evaluate the tongue's shape and size

- Look at the shape and size of the tongue.

- A normal tongue is typically symmetrical, with a moderate thickness.

- A swollen tongue may indicate fluid retention or dampness in the body.

- A thin or withered tongue may suggest a deficiency of qi or blood.

Step 4: Note any cracks or spots

- Check for cracks, spots, or other irregularities on the tongue's surface.

- Cracks may suggest a deficiency or dryness in the body.

- Spots or ulcers may indicate heat or toxicity in the body.

Step 5: Consider other characteristics

- Please consider other tongue characteristics, such as moisture level, texture, and movement.

- A dry tongue may suggest a deficiency of fluids in the body.

- A greasy or slimy tongue may indicate excess dampness or phlegm in the body.

- A stiff or trembling tongue may suggest an internal imbalance.

It's important to note that tongue diagnosis is just one part of the overall diagnostic process in TCM and should not be relied upon as a sole diagnostic tool. The interpretations of tongue characteristics in TCM may vary depending on the specific school of TCM or the practitioner's experience and expertise. It's essential to consult with a qualified and licensed TCM practitioner for accurate and reliable assessment and interpretation of tongue diagnosis findings.

Teeth Charting

Circadian360's
MERIDIAN TOOTH CHART

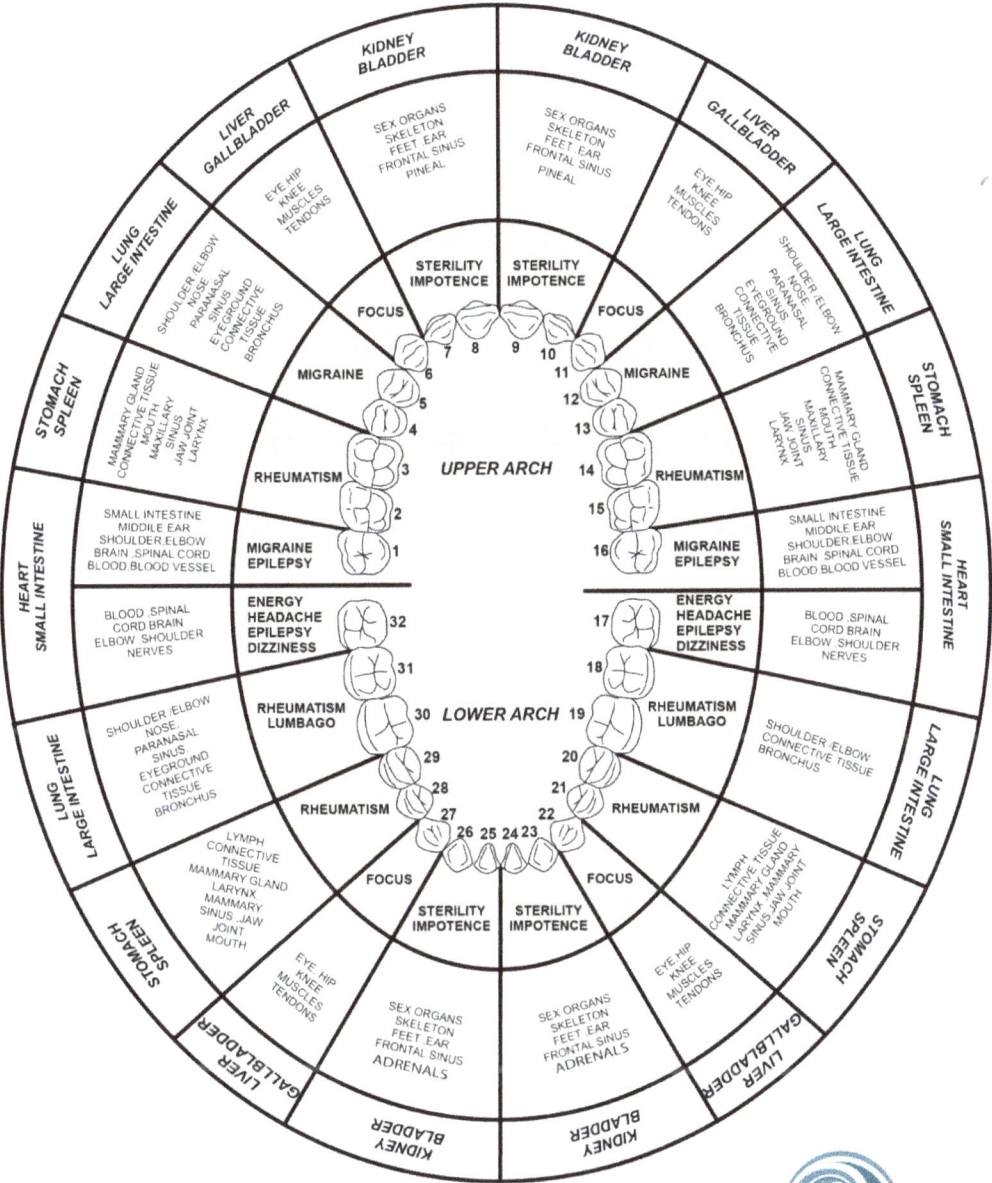

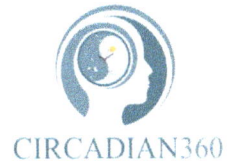

Teeth charting, on the other hand, is a system that associates specific teeth with various organs or body systems.

Also known as the Meridian Tooth Chart, this system is often used in alternative medicine, such as acupuncture, acupressure, and Traditional Chinese Medicine. It relies on the concept of meridians, which are believed to be energy channels connecting various body organs or tissues. According to this system, each tooth is thought to be connected to a specific meridian, and issues with the tooth may indicate imbalances or dysfunction in the associated meridian or organ. This process has been also known as dental meridian charting or tooth organ charting.

It's important to note that dental meridian charting is not recognized as a scientifically proven or accepted diagnostic tool in conventional dentistry or medicine. The associations between teeth and body parts in dental meridian charts are based on alternative or complementary theories and are not supported by mainstream scientific evidence. Therefore, it is crucial to approach dental meridian charting with caution and consult with qualified healthcare professionals for evidence-based and conventional dental and medical care.

Oil Pulling

Oil pulling is an ancient Ayurvedic practice believed to have originated in India over 3,000 years ago. It involves swishing oil, typically sesame or coconut oil, in the mouth for a period to improve oral health and overall well-being.

Here are step-by-step instructions for oil pulling at home:

1. **Choose an oil**: You can use organic coconut or olive oil. For maximum effectiveness, it's best to use cold-pressed, organic, and unrefined oils.
2. **Start with an empty stomach:** Oil pulling is typically done in the morning on an empty stomach before eating or drinking anything.

3. **Take about one tablespoon of oil into your mouth and swish it around.**
Do not swallow the oil, but move it around in your mouth, pulling and pushing it through your teeth and gums. Aim to do this for 15-20 minutes.

4. **Spit out the oil:** After the recommended time, spit out the oil into a trash can or disposable bag. Do not spit the oil into the sink or toilet. It can solidify and clog pipes.

5. **Rinse your mouth:** Rinse your mouth thoroughly with warm water to remove any remaining oil from your mouth.

6. **Brush and floss your teeth:** Follow up with brushing and flossing your teeth as you normally would to remove any residual oil and maintain good oral hygiene.

Best practices for oil pulling:

• Start with a smaller amount of oil (e.g., one teaspoon) if you are new to oil pulling, and gradually increase the amount as you become more comfortable with the process.

• Avoid swallowing the oil, as it may contain toxins and bacteria you are trying to remove from your mouth.

• Spit the used oil into a disposable bag or trash can, as it can solidify and clog drains, or make sure to spit it down the drain while hot water is running.

• Do not gargle or swallow the oil during the oil-pulling process, as this may reintroduce the toxins into your system.

• After oil pulling, it's essential to brush and floss your teeth to remove any remaining oil and maintain oral hygiene.

While there is limited scientific research specifically on combining activated charcoal and organic clove with organic coconut oil for oil pulling, both activated charcoal and organic clove have been studied for their potential medicinal benefits on the body.

These ingredients have been combined throughout ancient cultures to help in oral health:

- **Activated charcoal** is known for its adsorptive properties, which may help to trap and remove toxins and impurities from the mouth.
- **Organic clove**, on the other hand, has antimicrobial properties that may help to combat bacteria and promote oral health.
- **Coconut oil** is believed to have antibacterial properties. It may act as a carrier oil to help deliver the beneficial properties of activated charcoal and organic clove to the mouth during oil pulling. Use organic, cold pressed, unrefined, heaven free Coconut Oil if and whenever possible.

Remember that oil pulling should not be used as a substitute for professional medical or dental advice. It's always best to seek guidance from a qualified healthcare professional before incorporating new ingredients into your oil-pulling routine or oral hygiene practices. If you experience discomfort or adverse reactions, discontinue the practice and seek medical advice.

Benefits of Flossing

Flossing is a crucial oral hygiene practice with numerous dental health benefits. Some of the benefits of flossing include:

Plaque and food particle removal: Flossing helps remove plaque and food particles between the teeth and the gum line, where toothbrushes cannot reach. This helps prevent bacteria buildup, leading to tooth decay, gum disease, and bad breath.

Gum health: Flossing helps to clean the area between the teeth and gums, which can help prevent gum disease. Regular flossing can help to reduce inflammation and bleeding of the gums, which are early signs of gum disease.

Cavity prevention: By removing plaque and food particles, flossing helps to prevent the formation of cavities, especially in the areas between the teeth where cavities are common.

Fresh breath: Flossing helps to remove food particles and bacteria that can cause bad breath, helping to keep your breath fresh and clean.

The dangers of not regularly flossing can include:

Plaque buildup: Without regular flossing, plaque can build up between the teeth and along the gum line, leading to an increased risk of tooth decay and gum disease.

Gum disease: Poor oral hygiene, including lack of flossing, can lead to gum disease, which can cause symptoms such as red, swollen, and bleeding gums and eventually lead to tooth loss if left untreated.

Bad breath: Food particles and bacteria can remain trapped between the teeth without flossing, leading to bad breath.

Flossing has also been linked to heart disease and cardiovascular health. Some research suggests that there may be a correlation between gum disease and heart disease. This is because the bacteria from gum disease can enter the bloodstream and contribute to plaque formation in arteries, potentially leading to heart disease. Regular flossing and other good oral hygiene practices can help reduce gum disease risk and potentially lower heart disease risk.

Circadian360 CELLULAR DETOX PROTOCOL

Circadian360 Cellular Detox Protocol is a revolutionary program designed to help you optimize your health and wellness on a cellular level, through the ancient wisdom of the body clock and the modern science of intermittent fasting. An opportunity to reset and refresh yourself by supporting your five senses, this program is not just a diet, it's a lifestyle and wellness cleanse that will empower you to take control of all areas of your life!

The program is founded on the Nobel prize-winning research that supports the traditional healing methods of cultures like Ayurveda and Traditional Chinese Medicine, which have used the body clock for centuries to promote optimal health and longevity. By aligning with the natural rhythms of the earth, our solar system, and the universe, we can achieve greater physical, mental, and spiritual balance.

With the **Circadian360 Cellular Detox Protocol**, you'll discover a new level of vitality and energy as you naturally detoxify your body on a cellular level. You'll enjoy delicious, whole foods that nourish your body and mind, and learn how to incorporate intermittent fasting to supercharge your metabolism and optimize your weight loss.

In the context of food sensitivities and allergies, trigger foods are foods that can cause an adverse reaction in some people. This can include symptoms such as digestive issues, skin problems, respiratory issues, headaches, and more. Identifying and avoiding trigger foods can be important for individuals with food sensitivities or allergies, as it may help them maintain their health and well-being. The **Circadian360 Cellular Detox Protocol** can assist participants in identifying their trigger foods by systematically eliminating common allergens and then gradually reintroducing them. This process, especially when overseen by a healthcare professional, allows individuals to observe how their body responds to different foods. Please note that for individuals with severe allergies or sensitivities, it is crucial to undertake this process under the guidance of a qualified healthcare professional to ensure safety and proper support throughout the journey.

For beginners, it is recommended that you start with completing **Cycle 1: Circadian360 Parasite Cleanse - 14 Days**, before proceeding with **Cycle 2: Circadian360 Cellular Detox Tea - 30 Days**. For those who are more seasoned with similar lifestyle routines to the **Circadian360 Cellular Detox Protocol**, you may extend the duration of **Cycle 2: Circadian360 Cellular Detox Tea** for an additional 30-60 days. This means that upon completion of your initial **Cycle 2: Circadian360 Cellular Detox Tea - 30 Days**, you are able to assess your progress and may choose to continue your detox journey for another 30-60 Days. Beginners are encouraged to take Saturday's off (Do not drink your **Circadian360** teas on this day), while still adhering to the ***BEST DETOX PRACTICES*** on the weekends, eating only fiber-rich fruits and vegetables (raw and organic produce only, if possible!).

The **Circadian360 Cellular Detox Protocol** involves intermittent fasting, and for this reason, individuals should only consider and complete this protocol when they are able to refrain from overexertion, working out, going to the gym, lifting weights and/or raising their heart rates to elevated levels.

This protocol and the associated products and recommendations are not intended to diagnose, treat, cure, or prevent any disease. It's important to prioritize your health and safety. Before embarking on any new diet or wellness program, especially if you have underlying health conditions, we strongly encourage you to consult a licensed healthcare professional. Their expertise ensures that you make informed decisions tailored to your specific needs. Your well-being is paramount, and professional guidance can help you navigate this program effectively and safely.

How does it help to detox on a cellular level?

The **Circadian360 Cellular Detox Protocol** has been designed for success, as it dials in on the circadian rhythm to optimize mitochondrial health, focusing in on a key metabolite known as Nicotinamide Adenine Dinucleotide (NAD+).

NAD+ is considered a longevity molecule, and it unfortunately decreases with age. A co-enzyme that is found in all living cells, we need NAD+ for energy production, metabolic processes, mitochondrial function, inflammation, cell division, antioxidant defense, DNA repair, and of course, circadian rhythm health. With age, there is a decrease in NAD+ levels primarily due to increased oxidative stress and reduced antioxidant defense (as shown in PMID: 22848760); furthermore, some research suggests that excessive exposure to artificial blue light, especially at night, can interfere with circadian rhythms and potentially impact overall health, including NAD+ levels.

Exposure to blue light, especially from electronic devices like smartphones, tablets, and computers, can suppress the production of melatonin, a hormone that regulates our sleep-wake cycles. Disrupted sleep patterns can have a negative impact on overall health, potentially affecting NAD+ levels indirectly. Poor sleep can lead to cellular stress and inflammation, which may affect NAD+ metabolism and utilization.

The Circadian360 Cellular Detox Protocol allows individuals to raise their NAD+ levels naturally, guiding participants on a journey of circadian rhythm alignment, lowering inflammation, intermittent fasting, caloric awareness, encouraging energized exercise/movement and strategic reduction of artificial blue light consumption.

The protocol also centers around a plant-based diet, recognizing the abundant health benefits associated with consuming whole, plant-based foods. This dietary approach offers the body a wealth of essential nutrients, antioxidants, and phytochemicals that promote cellular health, repair, and overall well-being. This program encourages individuals to focus on consuming nutrient-dense foods from natural sources, while avoiding meat, dairy, soy, processed products and the overconsumption of seed oils high in omega-6 fatty acids.

Why should I follow this program?

The circadian rhythm is one of the biological rhythms that are crucial for regulating various bodily functions, including sleep, temperature control, and even some hormonal changes. These biological rhythms extend beyond sleep-wake cycles and significantly influence metabolism, heart rate, blood pressure and so much more. They even play a role in regulating blood sugar, cholesterol, mental health conditions, immune system function, DNA repair, and even the effectiveness of cancer treatments.

Just as professional athletes tend lose their expert abilities over time, our circadian rhythm becomes less efficient the older we get; moreover, due to both the overconsumption of electronic devices emitting blue light and late-night eating, we are finding a phenomenon where now younger people are living with less efficient circadian rhythms. This is known as "the flattening" of the circadian rhythm, and it was proven in 2017, through research conducted by Susan Hood and Shimon Amir in their paper "The aging clock: circadian rhythms and later life - PMID:28145903".

As we age, the body's circadian rhythm undergoes many changes including the dampening of the circadian hormones melatonin and cortisol, reduced circadian signaling through the eyes and brain, as well as shorter and more fragmented sleep cycles. Research is also finding that older people are now sleeping significantly less than younger individuals. This is primarily due to circadian system damage, as revealed in a 2004 study by Maurice M Ohayon and colleagues titled 'Meta-analysis of quantitative sleep parameters from childhood to old age in healthy individuals: developing normative sleep values across the human lifespan - PMID: 15586779'. This happens because our melatonin levels decrease with age, and older individuals produce a significantly less amount of melatonin than younger people. When we honor the fact that melatonin is also an anti-aging hormone, the strongest antioxidant, has powerful anti-inflammatory benefits, helps to regulate longevity, promotes cellular repair and has cardio and neuroprotective benefits, we can understand that lower melatonin levels eventually result in both less cellular repair and faster aging.

While many may think melatonin is simply related to sleep, it also supports apoptosis, autophagy, brain detoxing, bone health, immune health, fat burning and cognitive wellness/memory health. All this being said, fortunately, we are able to reverse damage done to our circadian rhythm, and this is exactly where the Circadian360 Cellular Detox Protocol finds itself appropriately positioned in your life.

Why does this program emphasize eliminating ALL artificial light sources after sunset?

With the rise of television, computers and now LED lights, in the span of less than 100 years, we've been unintentionally bombarding ourselves with toxic sources of light.

The blue light you see in the sky due to Rayleigh scattering, a phenomenon where shorter wavelengths scatter more easily, is related to the blue light emitted by LED (Light Emitting Diode) lights. Both types of blue light have a similar color appearance because they involve light in the blue part of the visible spectrum. The blue light in the sky is natural sunlight that has been scattered by the Earth's atmosphere, while LED lights are artificial sources containing blue light created using semiconductor technology. LED lights can be much more intense and concentrated compared to the relatively diffuse blue light from the sky. This intensity can have significant negatives affects upon our overall health.

The blue light from screens tricks the brain into thinking it's still daytime, suppressing melatonin production, a hormone that regulates our sleep-wake cycles, making it more challenging to fall asleep. Even with older tube-style televisions, staring at the TV screen for extended periods, especially late at night, contributed to sleep disruptions; moreover, depending on the television program, computer application, website, app, social media platform, texting service, and even your LED nightlights and household lightbulbs, the continual jolts of excitation and stimulation from these artificial light sources keep the brain engaged and alert.

So imagine, since the beginning of the 3rd Industrial Revolution, we have unintentionally been slowly reproducing offspring, generation after generation, to be born into a false blue light world powered by artificial lights, and in this 24/7 consumer casino, you pay not just with credit cards but also with your time on Earth and life-force.

It's okay that many of us didn't learn, know, or apply this knowledge prior to this moment, but it is now one's choice and responsibility to make the changes that are within their control.

It is time for us to upgrade our light to upgrade our life.

"..BUT I don't think blue light affects me because I watch my LED tv past 10pm and have no problem going to sleep. I even sleep with the tv shining on my face. Does this still apply to me?"

The Circadian360 Cellular Detox Protocol will certainly benefit you especially if you still find yourself waking up feeling tired and/or you get sleepy, fatigued, depressed, anxious or stressed throughout your days. With the constant stream of artificial light and mental stimulation, even when you're resting, you may not be entering into the deep REM (Rapid Eye Movement) state of sleeping that we need.

During the night, most people experience cycles of REM (Rapid Eye Movement) and non-REM sleep, including deep sleep and lighter stages of sleep. In REM sleep, our brains are highly active, often associated with vivid dreaming, while non-REM sleep consists of several stages, with deep sleep (or slow-wave sleep) being the most rejuvenating. Deep sleep is crucial for physical restoration, strengthening the immune system, and consolidating memories. Deep sleep, also known as slow-wave sleep, is essential for physical and mental restoration. It is often believed that the majority of deep sleep occurs earlier in the night, during the first half of the sleep period.

If you're not entering this deep state of rest and find yourself waking up frequently throughout the night, you're missing out on the essential physical and mental restoration that your body and mind require. Insufficient deep sleep can lead to impaired cognitive function, weakened immune response, increased stress levels, and a higher risk of chronic health conditions. Addressing these sleep issues is vital for your overall well-being and vitality.

Why is this a plant-based diet?

If the body is a car, the quality of fuel that one puts inside certainly matters, and just as we wash our cars to keep them clean, how often and when we get a checkup (self-assessment), oil change (detox) and/or need heavy service work (surgery) matters too.

It's crucial to recognize that food serves as the fuel for our cellular energy, nourishing our light body. This process of converting food into glucose is essential, especially for the brain, as it serves as a vital source of cellular energy. The speed at which food is converted to sugar and enters the bloodstream is referred to as the glycemic index(GI), measuring how quickly the carbohydrates in a particular food raise blood sugar levels.

The frequencies of our foods are interconnected with and influenced by the rhythms of the sun. When it comes to processed foods, the term "processed" generally refers to foods that have undergone various forms of manufacturing or refinement. These foods often contain added sugars, unhealthy fats, and other additives. The processing of food can remove or alter its natural fiber content, which plays a role in how quickly the carbohydrates are broken down and absorbed by the body.

Consuming processed foods, especially those with high glycemic indexes, can cause a rapid increase in blood sugar levels. This can put stress on the pancreas, which produces insulin to regulate blood sugar levels. If the pancreas is unable to produce enough insulin to compensate for the rapid spike in blood sugar, it can lead to various health issues, including insulin resistance and type 2 diabetes.

On the other hand, raw foods, such as fruits, vegetables, and whole grains, typically have a lower glycemic index because they contain more natural fiber and are digested more slowly. The slower digestion process allows for a more gradual release of glucose into the bloodstream, which helps maintain stable blood sugar levels and provides sustained energy.

This emphasis on consuming raw foods is not only beneficial for managing blood sugar levels but also for addressing three often overlooked factors in overall health: congestion, inflammation and mucus.

Why does the Circadian360 Cellular Detox Protocol encourage overnight intermittent fasting?

"Intermittent fasting means that you don't eat for a period of time each day or week. Intermittent fasting is any of the various meal timing schedules that cycle between voluntary fasting and non-fasting over a given period. Methods of intermittent fasting include alternate-day fasting, periodic fasting, and daily time-restricted feeding." - as defined by Mayo Clinic

If you're going from eating a diet heavy in animal meat, dairy, soy, refined carbohydrates, sugars and adopt the Circadian360 Cellular Detox Protocol plant-based diet that's packed with large amounts of high frequency fruits, vegetables and sprouted grains, you may see changes in several areas, including:

Reduced body weight.

Improved heart and vascular health.

Improved blood sugar control.

Reduced joint pain.

Improved bowel health and regularity.

Reduced cancer risk.

Intermittent fasting based on the circadian rhythm can be beneficial due to the natural alignment between our biological processes and the daily light-dark cycle. Our bodies have evolved to follow a pattern of activity and rest that corresponds to the availability of food and light during the day. By incorporating intermittent fasting into our routine, we can optimize this alignment and promote various health benefits.

Fasting, particularly overnight, allows our bodies to fully utilize the natural fasting period that occurs during sleep. During this time, the body gradually depletes its glycogen stores and transitions into a state called ketosis. In ketosis, the body starts breaking down stored fat to produce ketones, which serve as an alternative source of energy. This metabolic shift can support fat loss and improve insulin sensitivity.

When our bodies surpass the 13-hour fasting mark, several physiological changes occur. As the duration of fasting increases, the body's energy stores become further depleted, prompting a more significant reliance on fat oxidation. This can lead to increased autophagy, a cellular recycling process that helps remove damaged molecules and promotes cellular repair. Autophagy has also been associated with anti-aging effects and reduced risk of certain diseases.

Allowing the body to extended fasting periods can stimulate the production of growth hormones, which plays a crucial role in muscle recovery and growth, tissue repair, and overall metabolic health. Higher growth hormone levels can enhance fat burning, preserve muscle mass, and support cellular regeneration.

In addition to these metabolic and cellular benefits, intermittent fasting based on the circadian rhythm can help regulate hunger hormones, improve digestion, and promote a healthier relationship with food. It may also enhance mental clarity and focus, as the body becomes more efficient at utilizing energy sources during fasting periods.

Getting Started with the Circadian360 Cellular Detox Protocol

As circadian beings of light, our yearly cycle affords us two perfectly aligned opportunities to intentionally support ourselves in performing a safe, natural cleanse and detox. During these periods, we are provided with opportunities to reflect on the growth and losses of the previous season. It's a time to clear our body's pasture and prepare the soil for the upcoming season. We must till the body's soil, letting go of habits, relationships, environments, patterns, and thoughts that don't contribute to our growth. Please listen and weed them out! Don't be afraid to pull a weed that you thought was a flower growing, and sometimes, we don't realize the depth of a weed's prickly needles until we pull it out. Without this experience, how can we be prepared to identify and remove them in the future?

Through intentional planning, we sow the seeds for future harvests, consciously following through with our sustained daily efforts. In this, we are watering those seeds of directed intention and doing everything in our part to see them grow, fruit and provide us with a bounty in our lives, but we must remember: even when we do EVERYTHING in our part and to the best of our abilities…sometimes too much or too little rain, drought, planning, landscaping, effort can ruin a crop. This is natural, and we must embrace it as an integral part of life. We must not become defeated; rather, we mourn and let go, allowing us to find the blessings and joy within the grace of allowance that we once again have an opportunity for NEW growth. At this moment, we fall back on the tutelage, experience and training of our past seasons and move forward.

Every Circadian360 Cellular Detox Protocol cycle is a friendly reminder of your birthright to resetting, resting and recalibrating all areas of your life, and like time before, soon, an ascended clarification in your purpose will arise.

BEST DETOXING TIMES ACCORDING TO THE COSMIC CLOCK

The cosmic clock refers to the movement of celestial bodies such as the sun, moon, and planets.

Best Times to Parasite Cleanse: Winter & Summer Solstice

Best Times to Cellular Detox: Solar Aphelion & Perihelion

Best Times to Plant Seeds of Intention for Your Life:

   Pre-Fall August 15 - September 15;

   Pre-Spring Feb 15 - March 15

Step by Step Guide to Getting Started with the Circadian360 Cellular Detox Protocol

Step 1 - Upgrade Your Light & Upgrade Your Life! The first step is to 'Reset Your Body Clock & FREE YOURSELF from Artificial Light!' Begin your cellular reset by following the Circadian360 Pineal Decalcification recommendations and practices, to reduce your exposure to artificial light sources.

Step 2 - Establish Your Non-Negotiable Lifestyle Routine. Developing your non-negotiable, signature lifestyle routine that aligns with the body clock is a critical component of maintaining good health and wellness. It is also a great way of establishing the boundaries that you need for your optimum health and well-being.

Step 3 - Follow the Circadian360 Cellular Detox Protocol Daily Routine. Advanced participants may extend Cycle 2 for up to 30-60 days and/or until they are truly thriving in their light rhythm of life.

Step 4 Incorporate Circadian360 Herbal & Nutritional Support. Extensive research has indicated that any detoxification or lifestyle change strategy is significantly enhanced when it includes a thorough parasite cleanse. Often lurking within our bodies, these internal parasites can hinder the body's natural ability to cleanse and detoxify effectively. Once the human body undergoes a comprehensive parasite cleanse, it becomes more aligned and prepared to receive herbal support. These natural herbal remedies aid the body's inherent self-cleansing mechanisms, eliminating harmful elements and waste. Additionally, they play a crucial role in improving mitochondrial health, ensuring the body's energy centers are functioning optimally.

Cycle 1: Circadian360 Parasite Cleanse (14 Days)

Cycle 2: Circadian360 Cellular Detox Tea (30 Days)

Cycle 2 (optional): Circadian360 High Frequency Heavy Metal Flush (30 Days)

Cycle 2 (optional): Circadian360 Vegan Chocolate Mushroom Protein

Powder (30 Days)

Don't be afraid to use the provided Circadian360 support resources! Including the Circadian360 Cellular Detox Best Practices, the Circadian360 Cellular Detox Protocol offers you meaningful ways to take control of your health, internally and externally. Don't forget to take the time to do the foundational work to support your mental health, by practicing mindfulness, exercising and journaling.

Circadian360 Group Coaching with the Founder of Circadian360 - Step into a world of collective transformation with Circadian360 Group Detox Coaching, where individuals from diverse corners of the globe converge online under the nurturing guidance of Circadian360's author & program creator R.A. Massey. In this vibrant community, participants gain access to a treasure trove of Circadian360 resources. From Massey's entire library of previously published books in eBook format to direct messaging with fellow members and exclusive one-on-one conversations with Massey himself, the benefits are boundless. Engage in livestream classes, fireside chats with wellness and innovation luminaries, and be the first to explore new courses and literary works. Together, we cultivate a space where shared aspirations and collective wisdom become catalysts for personal growth. Embrace the power of community, embark on your detox journey, and let's thrive as one, rewriting our stories of wellness and vitality together.

Circadian360 Mindfulness & Manifestations Workbook - This workbook is not just a guide; it's an invitation to explore the inner landscapes of your soul. Rooted in the profound legacy of teachers like Venerable Ledi Sayadaw, S. N. Goenka, Jon Kabat-Zinn, Venerable Master Hsuan Hua, and the transformative guidance of mentors like Bill Brevoort, written and curated by R.A. Massey, the Circadian360 Mindfulness & Manifestations Workbook serves as your companion on the profound journey of self-discovery. Imagine tending to your spirit's zen garden, nurturing it with mindfulness, Vipassana, meditation, and yoga – tools to till the soil of your mind. As you delve into the transformative exercises, guided by the light of your awareness, you'll unearth the roots of past traumas, navigate tangled habits, and plant the seeds of newfound wisdom. Just as a master landscaper tends to a garden, this workbook empowers you to cultivate your mind deliberately, addressing the shadows, uprooting the weeds, and allowing the blossoms of intention to flourish.

Circadian360 Journal - The Circadian360 Journal is not just a blank canvas; it's a sanctuary for your thoughts and dreams, a sacred space where accountability meets self-care. With each entry, you embark on a transformative journey, reflecting on the tapestry of your day under the gentle glow of the moon. Here, amidst the blank pages, you become the architect of your future, shaping your aspirations, pondering your challenges, and celebrating your triumphs. This journal isn't just about writing; it's about becoming, allowing your thoughts to take flight, guiding you toward your best self. Embrace the power of introspection, let the ink flow, and watch as your words become the foundation upon which your dreams flourish.

STEP 1: The Pineal Gland Decalcification

Welcome to Circadian360's Pineal Decalcification Guide, a critical response to the alarming trend observed in younger generations: a rapid increase in pineal gland calcification.

While calcification naturally occurs with age, studies reveal a concerning shift: Many individuals now exhibit pineal calcifications at an early age, disrupting the delicate balance of melatonin production, our body's sleep regulator.

This calcification, a potential consequence of constant exposure to artificial blue light and circadian disruption, is not just a natural part of aging—it's a warning sign. We've witnessed cases where people in their 70s have minimal calcifications, and yet, now we are finding younger individuals developing them. Melatonin, the hormone produced by the pineal gland that's essential for quality sleep and overall health, is at stake. Melatonin is also an anti-aging hormone, the strongest antioxidant, has powerful anti-inflammatory benefits, helps to regulate longevity, promotes cellular repair and has cardio and neuroprotective benefits

The urgency of this matter cannot be overstated. This guide isn't just a solution; it's a necessity.

Join the Circadian360 community in this vital endeavor to preserve your melatonin production, protect your pineal gland, and secure a healthier future, unburdened by the shadows of premature aging and disrupted sleep.

Realign Your Body Clock with the Sun

Waking up just before sunrise and basking in the natural morning light helps synchronize your internal body clock with the Earth's natural rhythm. This practice, rooted in our evolutionary history, triggers the production of serotonin, enhancing mood and energy. The pineal gland is activated specifically by the blue light of the the morning sun when it is between 450-500nm wavelength, signaling for the suppression of melatonin production. Roughly 12 hours later, as the sun begins to set and the wavelengths of light decrease, melatonin production begins to increase, leading to drowsiness and sleep. Going to bed no later than 10 p.m. ensures you get the recommended hours of restorative sleep, allowing your body to fully engage in its nightly repair and rejuvenation processes. Embracing this harmonious cycle not only supports a healthy circadian rhythm and melatonin production but also promotes overall well-being, mental clarity, and emotional balance.

Intentional Acts of Grounding

In our modern world we are constantly saturated with harmful electromagnetic frequencies (EMFs), emitted by electronic devices, and due to this bombardment, our bodies often struggle to maintain their natural balance. Scientifically rooted in the Schumann Resonance, the Earth's natural frequency is approximately 7.83 Hz, and grounding acts as a bridge connecting us to this vital rhythm. Research suggests that grounding allows us to absorb the Earth's electrons, helping to neutralize free radicals and reduce inflammation, promoting cellular stability and overall health within the body. The umbrella effect is a phenomenon observed when grounding effectively shields the body from EMFs, and it underscores the profound impact of this practice. By intentionally grounding ourselves, we tap into the Earth's subtle energies, rebalancing and realigning our bodies, fostering improved sleep, enhanced immunity, and a deep sense of vitality.

Illuminate Your Evening by Candlelight

Embrace your evenings with the flickering warmth of candles, a decisive step toward reclaiming your sleep sanctuary. Choose wisely, opting for candles sourced from natural, non-toxic ingredients, free from harmful fragrances. Rediscover the ancestral wisdom of incorporating gas lamps, mirroring the gentle glow our predecessors relied on. Urgency lies in these intentional choices: we must disrupt the invasion of artificial lights, forging a sanctuary conducive to deep, restorative sleep. Embracing this urgent shift not only safeguards your circadian rhythm but also nurtures your well-being, fostering a sacred space where tranquility reigns and vitality thrives.

Harmful Ingredients and Fragrances to Avoid:

Paraffin Wax: Derived from petroleum, it releases harmful chemicals when burned.

Lead Wicks: Can release toxic lead fumes when the candle burns.

Artificial Fragrances: Often contain phthalates, which are linked to hormone disruption.

Benzene and Toluene: VOCs (Volatile Organic Compounds) found in some candle fragrances, associated with respiratory issues.

Acetone: Another VOC found in fragrances, potentially harmful when inhaled.

Soy Wax: Though now considered to be a renewable resource, this candle still emits toxins though fewer than the others mentioned. Also soy is an endocrine disruptor, and inhaling soy may still be contributing towards the overall balance and/or imbalance of your endocrine system.

<u>Safer Alternatives to Consider:</u>

Beeswax: Naturally filtered, releases negative ions that can improve indoor air quality.

Cotton or Wood Wicks: Lead-free and safer for the environment.

Essential Oils: Natural scents derived from plants, offering various therapeutic benefits.

Non-GMO Vegetable-based Dyes: For colored candles, opt for natural, plant-based dyes.

<u>Additional Tips</u>:

Look for candles labeled as "phthalate-free" and "lead-free wicks."

If exploring gas lamps, ensure proper ventilation and consult with professionals to ensure safe usage.

Reducing Artificial Light Exposure

The blue light from your phone is the false blue light of the sky!

The blue light you see in the sky due to Rayleigh scattering is actually related to the blue light emitted by LED (Light Emitting Diode) lights. Both types of blue light have a similar color appearance because they involve light in the blue part of the visible spectrum. The blue light in the sky is natural sunlight that has been scattered by the Earth's atmosphere, while LED lights are artificial sources containing blue light created using semiconductor technology. LED lights can be much more intense and concentrated compared to the relatively diffuse blue light from the sky. This intensity can have significant negatives affects upon our overall health.

What ends up happening is that the blue light from screens tricks the brain into thinking it's still daytime, suppressing melatonin production and making it more challenging to fall asleep. Even with older tube-style televisions, staring at the TV screen for extended periods, especially late at night, contributed to sleep disruptions; moreover, contingent upon the television program, computer application, website, app, social media platform, texting service and/or even your LED nightlights and household lightbulbs, the continual jolts of excitation and stimulation from these artificial light sources keeps the brain engaged and alert.

LED lights can be found in various places in our homes, and some of these locations might disrupt natural nighttime darkness. Here are common places where LED lights are used in households- Household bulbs, nightlights, flashlights, electronics (computers, laptops, smartphones, tablets, televisions), kitchen appliances, garden and patio lights, smart home devices.

To minimize the disruption of natural nighttime darkness, consider using warm white or amber-colored LED bulbs, especially in areas where you spend time in the evening. Additionally, using curtains or blinds to block outdoor light sources and turning off unnecessary electronic devices can help create a darker and more sleep-friendly environment at night.

Consider investing in blue light screen shields for your electronic devices, as well as blue light blocking glasses to wear at night. These investments in your health today may have significant, long-term benefits that can be appreciated years down the line.

STEP 2: Establish Your Non-Negotiable Lifestyle Routine

Answer The Following Questions Before You Begin

First thing - both designing and keeping the discipline to follow YOUR non-negotiable, daily plan that fits your lifestyle is the only way to see change. Nobody can live your life like you do, and the first step to unlocking your greatness is setting the boundaries of what your light body will and won't do during the 24-hour cycle. Many of us have never truly set boundaries for ourselves in many areas of our lives so developing a lifestyle routine may initially be daunting …but once you establish a true, unwavering foundation for yourself…the ascension of your soul, physical, mental, emotional bodies will both feel and be so rewarding!

Developing your non-negotiable lifestyle routine that aligns with the body clock is a critical component of maintaining good health and wellness. To support optimal health, answer these questions to help structure YOUR Circadian360 Daily Routine:

What time are you going to bed every night?

Maintain a regular sleep schedule: Going to bed and waking up at the same time every day can help regulate your internal clock and improve sleep quality. Irregular sleep patterns can disrupt the body's natural rhythms, leading to fatigue, mood swings, and other health issues.

Circadian360 recommends sleeping for 7+ hrs/night. Remember - Stop eating 3 hours before bed, and stop drinking liquids two hours before bed. Eating 3 hours before bed also may inhibit REM (Rapid Eye Movement) stage of sleep.

What time is breakfast, lunch and dinner? When will you grocery shop for the ingredients needed to prepare your meals for the week and/or day?

Eat in accordance with the body clock: Eating the main meal during the day and avoiding heavy meals late at night can help regulate metabolism and digestion. The digestive system is more active during the day, and eating late at night can interfere with the body's natural processes.

When not adhering to the detox protocol, eating a fresh, lefty green salad with vegetables is the best wellness hack to start your day. Save your fruit and/or fruit smoothies for early afternoon, to give your body a nourishing boost of nature's candy, to help fuel your energy until early evening; moreover, avoiding eating too many fruits in the evening, as we want to bring down our energy levels to prepare for a proper night's rest.

Dedicating, in advance, days and times for shopping and meal preparation allows you not to be inundated with spending future days of productivity or rest bogged down trying to figure out what to eat because you're too bored or busy. Bad dietary habits and crunch hunger decisions arise when we haven't adequately prepared ourselves for the moment in advance,

What time(s) are you getting sunlight and for how long?

Expose yourself to natural light: Natural light exposure during the day can help regulate the internal clock. Spending time outside for at least 30 minutes a day can help regulate the body's natural rhythms and improve overall health. The sun is also anabolic meaning it increases mitochondrial health and function, further supporting metabolic and hormonal health, muscle recovery, motivation and mood overall.

Circadian360 recommends spending 1-2+ hours a day in nature.

When are you getting in light movement during your day?

Incorporate regular light movement into your routine: Movement is essential for good health and can help regulate the internal clock. Try to go for outdoor walks, at the same time every day, to support the body's natural rhythms.

Walking outdoors for 1-2+ hours a day fulfills light movement and our daily sunlight requirement!

What time(s) will you stop using electronic devices?

Minimize exposure to artificial light at night: Exposure to artificial light at night can disrupt the body's natural rhythms. Avoid using electronic devices before bedtime and use blackout curtains to minimize exposure to external light sources.

<u>This program recommends that you strive to stop looking at screens AT LEAST 1 hour before bed.</u>

Incorporating these practices into your daily routine can help support the body's natural rhythms and optimize overall health and wellness. By aligning your lifestyle with the body clock, you can experience improved sleep quality, increased energy, and better overall health.

STEP 3: Follow the Circadian360 Cellular Detox Protocol Daily Routine

Circadian360 Cellular Detox Protocol DAILY ROUTINE

SUNRISE ILLUMINATIONS & BREAKING FAST WITH GRATITUDE - Honoring the Mind + Body + Spirit through Intentional Gratitude & Self Care.

A mindful morning ritual invites us to become the architects of our own well-being, building a foundation of intention and mindfulness that sustains us through the day's demands. It reminds us that every moment, whether spent in quiet reflection or active engagement, holds the potential for mindfulness— a gift we unwrap, through awareness, each day. By embracing these morning rituals, we embark on a journey where mindfulness intertwines with intention, unveiling the boundless beauty that resides within and around us.

Scientific research has begun to shed light on the profound impact of certain morning rituals on our physical and mental well-being. Stepping outside, barefoot, to allow your eyes to greet the gentle rays of the rising sun- these morning rituals, the seeds planted in the fertile soil of our minds and lives, ripple into our daily existence, reminding us of the importance of embracing the present moment. These rituals become a canvas upon which we paint the hues of our aspirations, cultivating a daily practice of mindfulness that transforms the ordinary into the extraordinary.

4a- 7a

- Wake Up
- Gratitudes, Affirmations & Intention Setting
- Meditation, Prayers & Tea Ceremony
- Physical Activity
- Family or Self-Care Time
- (Optional with Cycle 2 - Circadian360 High Frequency Heavy Metal Flush. Take immediately upon waking / rising from rest with 16oz water.)

What the Science Tells Us:

5 am - 7 am: The Large Intestine Hour

Body Functions: Large intestine detoxification, elimination, and hydration

Chinese Meridians: Large Intestine (LI1)

Things to Do: Drink plenty of water, practice gentle stretching exercises, avoid late-night snacks

Things to Avoid: Excessive consumption of alcohol, spicy or fatty foods, negative thoughts

7a - 11a

- Circadian360 Parasite Cleanse Tea or Cellular Detox Tea
- Vegetable & Non-Meat Protein Breakfast - NO FRUITS!
- Drink 6 cups of water (approximately 48oz) with hand-squeezed key limes

(2-4), limes (1-2) or lemons (1-2). You have the full 3-hours to drink your water and you DO NOT have to consume all 48oz at once.

- Remember - No Fruits before 11a!

What the Science Tells Us:

7 am - 9 am: The Stomach Hour

Body Functions: Stomach detoxification, nutrient absorption, and energy production

Chinese Meridians: Stomach (ST36)

Things to Do: Eat a healthy breakfast, practice gentle exercises, avoid skipping meals

Things to Avoid: Eating heavy or greasy foods, drinking too much caffeine, excessive mental stress

9 am - 11 am: The Pancreas Hour

Body Functions: Pancreatic detoxification, hormone regulation, and blood sugar control

Chinese Meridians: Spleen (SP3)

Things to Do: Eat a healthy breakfast, practice moderate exercises, take a walk in the sun

Things to Avoid: Skipping breakfast, eating sugary or processed foods, rushing or overworking

MIDDAY - PEAK PERFORMANCE - How are you maximizing your moments on this day? How are you being in service to others?

There's no amount of words offered that can compare to when your day is either full of green lights and/or you're rested, prepared and/or present enough to not let the yellow and red lights knock you off balance; however, what happens when they do?

Consider doing a random act of kindness for someone else, when your day isn't going quite right. Holding the door for someone, volunteering and/or donating to a charity is always a great way to remember that even though it may be raining on your parade, you can always be the sunshine in someone else's day and life. Somehow, being kind, generous and extending grace to others makes us feel better, but remember to not give more than you are able to give.

11a - 5p

- Plant-based Lunch (Optional - Circadian360 Vegan Chocolate Mushroom Protein Powder)
- Drink 6 cups of water (approximately 48oz) with hand-squeezed key limes (2-4), limes (1-2) or lemons (1-2). You have the full 3-hours to drink your water and you DO NOT have to consume all 48oz at once.

SNACK OPTIONS FOR SHORT ENERGY BURST:

Eat one to two servings of high fiber fruit and/or 1 Handful of Raw Nuts (Walnuts, Almonds, Pecans or Brazil Nuts). Do not mix fruits! Examples: One (1) to Two (2) Red Grapefruits or One (1) to Two (2) Apples. Avoid fruit juices and smoothies! Read more about why in both the Foods to Avoid & FAQ sections found later in the Circadian36 Cellular Detox Protocol.

What the Science Tells Us:

11 am - 1 pm: The Heart Hour

Body Functions: Heart detoxification, blood circulation, and emotional regulation

Chinese Meridians: Heart (HE8)

Things to Do: Take a break, practice relaxation techniques, express gratitude and joy

Things to Avoid: Overworking, excessive mental stress, consuming caffeinated beverages

1 pm - 3 pm: The Small Intestine Hour

Body Functions: Small intestine detoxification, nutrient absorption, and digestion

Chinese Meridians: Small Intestine (SI5)

Things to Do: Eat a healthy lunch, practice moderate exercises, take a break from work

Things to Avoid: Eating too quickly, consuming heavy or greasy foods, skipping meals

3 pm - 5 pm: The Bladder Hour

Body Functions: Bladder detoxification, fluid regulation, and hormone production

Chinese Meridians: Bladder (BL66)

Things to Do: Drink plenty of water, take a short nap or rest, practice relaxation techniques

Things to Avoid: Drinking too much caffeine, holding urine for too long, overexertion

MOON REFLECTIONS & RESTING WHEN WESTING - Pour into YOUR Cup. Restore Energy for the Next Sunrise.

In ancient Egyptian mythology, the west was associated with the realm of the dead and the setting sun. The east, on the other hand, was associated with life and rebirth because it was where the sun rose. Applying the concept of "westing" from ancient Egyptian beliefs to our modern lives as a way to end our days in reflection and preparation for a new day can be a meaningful and symbolic practice.

While the dawn invites us to set intentions and embrace positivity, the dusk beckons us to delve into deeper self-reflection. Reflect on the events, experiences, and emotions of the day. Consider both the positive and challenging aspects of your day. This is akin to the ancient Egyptians' belief in transitioning from life to the afterlife, where they reviewed their deeds.

By allocating time at the end of the day, week, month, season, and year for self-reflection and assessment, you create pockets of wisdom. These moments of retrospective contemplation offer insights that pave the way for growth and evolution throughout your forthcoming days and seasons.

5p - 7p

- Physical Activity
- Family or Self-Care Time
- Plant-Based Dinner (BEFORE Sunset)
- *Optional:* Drink 4 or more cups of water (approximately 32oz) with hand-squeezed key limes (2-4), limes (1-2) or lemons (1-2).

What the Science Tells Us:

5 pm - 7 pm: The Kidney Hour (continued)

Chinese Meridians: Kidney (KI10)

Things to Do: Drink plenty of water, practice gentle exercises, take a short break to rest your eyes

Things to Avoid: Excessive consumption of caffeine or alcohol, working too intensely, holding onto negative emotions.

7p - 10p

- Physical Activity
- Family or Self-Care Time
- Read
- Shadow Work & Journaling
- Sleep

Wind down tips:

Stop eating three hours before bed. (7p)

Stop drinking liquids two hours before bed. (8p)

Stop looking at screens 1 hour before bed. (9p)

Sleep (Listen to Solfeggio frequencies) (10p)

What the Science Tells Us:

7 pm - 9 pm: The Pericardium Hour

Body Functions: Pericardium detoxification, emotional regulation, and circulation

Chinese Meridians: Pericardium (P8)

Things to Do: Practice self-care, spend time with loved ones, do something enjoyable

Things to Avoid: Overworking, excessive stress, skipping meals or snacks

9 pm - 11 pm: The Triple Burner Hour

Body Functions: Triple Burner detoxification, hormone regulation, and metabolism

Chinese Meridians: Triple Burner / San Jiao (SJ6)

Things to Do: Have a light dinner, wind down with calming activities, spend quality time with loved ones

Things to Avoid: Eating heavy or greasy foods, watching TV or using electronic devices before bed, overthinking

STEP 4: Incorporate Circadian360 Herbal & Nutritional Support

Research has shown that no detox and/or full lifestyle change is beneficial without addressing the potential internal parasites that are living in our bodies. Once an individual has completed a parasite cleanse, their body is more aligned and prepared to proceed with receiving herbal support to help in the body's natural abilities to self-cleanse and detoxify/eliminating harmful elements and waste. This is why Circadian360's Cellular Detox Protocol is broken down into 2 distinct cycles.

Complete your Cycle 1: Circadian360 Parasite Cleanse - 14 Days, BEFORE proceeding to the Cycle 2: Circadian360 Cellular Detox Tea - 30 Days. Only when your Parasite Cleanse has been completed should you begin Cycle 2's Cellular Detox Tea. Due to the nature of the included herbs being so powerful, do NOT consume the

Parasite Cleanse Tea and the Cellular Detox Tea at the same time and/or during the same 14 Day period. This ensures that your body is properly supported during each flush, without causing strain, exhaustion and discomfort upon your digestive system. During Cycle 2, you are encouraged to begin incorporating the Circadian360 High Frequency Heavy Metal Flush and Circadian360 Vegan Chocolate Mushroom Protein Powder into your daily routines, and you are encouraged to continue using both of them until your cycle supply runs out.

CYCLE 1 - Parasite Cleanse Tea - 14 Days

Experience a transformative cleanse with our Parasite Cleanse, a potent blend meticulously crafted to rid your body of unwanted invaders. Infused with the power of nature's defenders, this cleanse features a comprehensive mix of ingredients designed to target and eliminate parasites. This cleanse not only purges invaders but also nourishes your body, leaving you feeling revitalized. Trust in the potency of nature and embark on your journey to a healthier, parasite-free you.

Follow the directions on your Circadian360 Parasite Cleanse, for instructions on how to successfully complete your cleanse.

CYCLE 2 - Cellular Detox Tea - 30 Days

Once you have completed the Cycle 1 - Circadian360 Parasite Cleanse, unlock the secrets of vibrant health with the specially crafted Circadian360 Cellular Detox Tea, expertly curated to nourish your body and promote overall well-being. Harnessing the power of nature's finest ingredients, each sip of this exquisite blend is a step towards hormonal balance, weight loss, thyroid support, blood cleansing, liver detoxification, and memory enhancement. Based on extensively researched botanicals, this tea is more than a beverage; it's a holistic approach to rejuvenating your body from the inside out.

Each sip of the Circadian360 Cellular Detox Tea is a step toward holistic health and vitality. Crafted with care and backed by scientific research, this tea is your natural ally in the journey towards a healthier, balanced, and rejuvenated you.

ADDITIONAL DETOX SUPPORT

CYCLE 2 – High Frequency Heavy Metal Flush (30 Days)

Upon completion of Cycle 1 - Parasite Cleanse, discover the power of nature's finest detoxifying agents in the Circadian360 High Frequency Heavy Metal Flush with Chlorella & Spirulina. Carefully crafted to shield your body against the harmful effects of heavy metals and environmental toxins, this potent blend of Chlorella and Spirulina offers a natural and scientifically backed solution for a thorough detoxification process.

Ingredients:

Chlorella: Rich in chlorophyll, Chlorella binds to heavy metals like mercury, lead, and cadmium, aiding in their elimination from the body. Studies have shown Chlorella's ability to reduce heavy metal toxicity significantly.

Spirulina: Packed with antioxidants like phycocyanin, Spirulina supports the body's natural detoxification pathways. Its high content of protein and essential amino acids promotes overall cellular health.

The Circadian360 High Frequency Heavy Metal Flush with Chlorella & Spirulina is your natural defense against environmental toxins. Backed by rigorous scientific research, this powerful blend ensures your body's natural detoxification pathways are fortified, allowing you to lead a healthier, toxin-free life.

CYCLE 2 - MEAL SUPPORT - Vegan Chocolate Mushroom Protein Powder (30 Days)

Upon completion of the Cycle 1 - Parasite Cleanse, crafted to fuel your body and elevate your mind, this unique blend combines the richness of vegan protein with the therapeutic power of wild-harvested Lion's Mane, Reishi, and Chaga mushrooms. Boosted with even more power with organic Reishi Mushroom Powder, every scoop is a celebration of holistic nourishment, providing unparalleled support for your physical and mental well-being.

Key Ingredients:

Lion's Mane: Known as the "smart mushroom," Lion's Mane supports brain health, enhancing cognitive function and promoting focus and clarity.

Reishi: Revered as the "mushroom of immortality," Reishi boosts the immune system, reduces stress, and supports overall vitality.

Chaga: Packed with antioxidants and immune-boosting properties, Chaga supports cellular health and helps combat oxidative stress.

The Circadian360 Cellular Detox Protocol's Best Practices

Our mitochondria are the heart of metabolic health. Every reaction in the human body is dependent on their health and function. The gradual changes that occur while completing the Circadian360 Cellular Detox Protocol have been consciously chosen as a guide to help support the optimization of the human being's mitochondria.

FIX MICRO-NUTRIENT DEFICIENCIES

Micro-nutrient deficiencies can also be harming your metabolic health. Use a food journal and nutrition tracker to see what nutrients your diet may be deficient in.

Asking your physician and/or health practitioner for assistance in both getting a mineral and nutrient analysis done, as well as a review of the results will also provide beneficial in deterring your specific dietary needs on a cellular level.

A great way to find out your current mineral count is to invest in having a hair tissue mineral analysis (HTMA) done. HTMA is a safe and non-invasive pathology test that measures the levels and comparative ratios of nutrient and toxic minerals found in hair. HTMA is one of the most valuable screening tools available in preventative health care.

Contact Circadian360 to have your HTMA testing done, in addition to a 1:1 consultation with R.A. Massey, author and creator of Circadian360, to discuss test results and healthy recommendations for moving forward.

LOWER STRESS WITH LIFE HACKS

- Spend 1-2 hours a day in nature, and practice the act of grounding
- Stop looking at screens at least 1 hour before bed.
- Wear blue-light blocking glasses after sunset
- Sunday's are for meal prepping, weekly planning and intention setting
- Listen to Solfeggio frequencies / binaural beats, especially while sleeping

SLEEP

- Your body needs to achieve a drop in temperature in order to get into deep sleep. This is why sleeping is much harder in the summer time when it's hot and humid. Keep your room at a lower temperature. 65 F is the most optimal for sleep.
- Keep your room as dark as possible. Turn off all the lights.
- Any light in your room will interfere with your sleep quality.
- Sleep 7+ hrs/night, gradually treating yourself to more than 7 hours consistently, whenever possible.

MANAGE EMOTIONS WITHOUT EATING FOOD

- Find consistent eating windows that work for you, and eat only when you're hungry; however, before you do eat, always ask yourself…

- *Am I hungry or am I bored?*
- *How will this food make me feel? (Energized or tired)*
- *Is there a lean protein source in this food?*
- *Could I go for a jog after eating this? (If not then you ate too much)*

- Walk after meals. Stop eating 3 hours before bed. Stop drinking liquids two hours before bed.

Remember - this journey is NOT about giving up some of your favorite foods forever; rather, the journey is about control and redefining a healthy balance for your long-term health!

PHYSICAL MOVEMENT

- Sprinting 3-5x / Week - Sprinting is a fitness hack with a big return on investment . Short 6-10 second sprints will increase fat loss, reduce stress, improve heart health and improve metabolic health.
- Start walking outdoors! Strive for 5-7k steps each day, and gradually increase to 10k+ steps!
- Finish working out 3 hours before bed.

STAY HYDRATED: DRINK WATER WITH MAGNESIUM!

Hydrate with plenty of spring water and not purified or distilled water. Natural spring water derives its mineral content from the geological formations it passes through.

These minerals, including calcium, magnesium, and potassium, contribute to the water's taste and potential health benefits. These minerals can support various bodily functions, from bone health to electrolyte balance.

It is crucial to stay hydrated while detoxing, as toxins and waste are being eliminated from the body. Drinking at least 10-12 cups (8oz each) of water or 1 gallon of spring water daily is recommended. The elimination of toxins can cause various symptoms such as skin rashes, acne, constipation, bad breath, night sweats, and headaches. Drinking ample water will help flush out these toxins and prevent their reabsorption, supporting the body's natural waste-removing mechanisms and promoting overall well-being.

Something to know: Whether your goal is losing fat or building muscle, hydration is the secret key, but what many may not be aware of is that salts and electrolytes help the absorption process so that the water isn't simply released through sweat and frequent urination.

The cell has a membrane around it, and in order to get water to the cell, magnesium is needed. So even though you are drinking more water, if you're not drinking quality water and/or still feeling drained, having frequent urination, low energy and/or shaky muscles, consider incorporating more salt into your diet; however, NOT ALL SALTS ARE THE SAME!

The common table salt is actually a dangerous salt, and the human body needs premium, natural sea salt as it is provided in nature, as it contains the magnesium and all other minerals the body requires from water. The best sea salts recommended:

Celtic Salt - Celtic salt is a treasure trove of minerals and boasts a unique pH balance that distinguishes it within the world of salts. Its distinctive composition includes a remarkable variety of trace minerals and electrolytes, resulting in a tapestry of flavors and benefits. With its intriguing **pH balance of 8.14**, it's mineral-rich profile boasts a captivating array of essential elements, trace minerals, and electrolytes, forming a harmonious symphony within the salt. With a **sodium chloride content of 88%**, Celtic salt distinguishes itself from conventional table salts that often comprise a higher percentage of sodium chloride.

Himalayan Salt - Renowned for its remarkable characteristics, Himalayan salt emerges as a truly exceptional mineral-rich option. Exhibiting distinctive attributes, including a treasure trove of essential trace minerals and electrolytes, as well as a **pH balance of 7.0 to 7.5**, Himalayan salt presents a unique mineral composition. With approximately **98% sodium chloride and an intriguing 2% comprising an array of naturally occurring trace minerals**, this salt possesses an intriguing contrast to conventional table salts. The allure of Himalayan salt lies not only in its mineral content but also in its captivating pale pink hue, a testament to its origin and the ancient sea beds from which it's sourced.

Hawaiian Alaea Salt - An exquisite coarse salt celebrated for its distinct qualities, including a naturally lower sodium content, elevated levels of trace minerals and electrolytes, and a remarkable **pH balance of 9.37**. This salt boasts a **sodium chloride content of 81%**, accompanied by an impressive **19% comprised of an array of 80 naturally present trace minerals**. These attributes set it apart from conventional table salts, which often consist of up to 99% sodium chloride. Red alaea is also rich in iron oxides, which makes for a great digestible form of dietary iron, in addition to being a minor source of copper. The coarse Alaea Red Sea Salt stands as a tribute to the extraordinary landscapes of Hawaii, embodying the essence of baked red Alaea clay derived from within the intricate layers of lava rocks. Traditionally, Hawaiians use Alaea in healing rituals and ceremonies to cleanse, purify and bless tools and canoes.

Based on pH, sodium chloride content and both percentage and amount of naturally present trace minerals, **Hawaiian Alaea Salt** is a perfect sea salt right from the USA. The island of Hawai'i is also not facing a shortage of red alaea or access to sea salt! Let us encourage more use of this salt, potentially boosting an industry for our youth, brothers, sisters, aunties, uncles and elders living on the Hawaiian Islands!

As summer heat causes the human body to sweat more, be even more mindful of your electrolyte intake. Also, consider choosing one of these high quality sea salts and consuming a pinch just before and after your exercise workouts.

INTERMITTENT FASTING

Fasting based on the circadian rhythm involves timing your meals to align with your body's natural 24-hour cycle. The goal is to optimize your digestion, metabolism, and energy levels by eating during the hours when your body is best able to process food and giving it a break during the hours when it needs to focus on repair and restoration.

Here are some general guidelines for fasting based on the circadian rhythm:

<u>Start with a 10-hour fast</u>: Aim to finish eating your last meal of the day by 7 or 8 pm, and then fast for 10 hours until breakfast the next morning. This gives your body time to fully digest your food and rest before starting the digestive process again.

<u>Gradually increase the fasting window</u>: As individuals extend their cycles, depending on one's personal goals and preferences, the fasting window may gradually be increased from 10 to up to 12-16 hours. Consider treating yourself to an extended fast, to allow your body to reach autophagy (as outlined in this section).

<u>Time your meals</u>: Try to eat during the daylight hours when your body is naturally more active and in need of fuel. This means having breakfast soon after waking up, having lunch around midday, and having dinner before the sun sets.

<u>NO late-night snacking</u>: Eating too close to bedtime can disrupt your sleep and interfere with your body's natural repair and restoration processes.

<u>…again…STAY HYDRATED</u>: Drink plenty of water, and consider incorporating herbal teas and infused waters to keep you hydrated and support your body's natural detoxification processes.

While every human body is slightly different, here is a general timeline of what happens when we are intermittent fasting; moreover, this is why this program encourages you to try to extend the hours between dinner and breakfast when possible. If and/or when you choose to do an **extended fast** for more than an overnight period, you are allowing the body to truly active it's natural cellular detoxification mechanisms.

4-8 Hours

Stomach is empty Blood sugars fall & insulin is not being produced

12 Hours

Consumed food has been burnt off

Digestive system goes to sleep Human Growth Hormone (HGH) begins to increase

14 Hours

Body begins to use stored fat as energy

HGH production ramps up

16-18 Hours

Fat burning ramps up & HGH production skyrockets

24 Hours

Autophagy begins (cell repair & cleaning)

Stored glycogen is emptied

Ketones released to blood stream (ketogenesis)

36-48 Hours

Autophagy increased 300%

Immune system resets and regenerates

Entering deep ketosis

60-72 Hours

Autophagy reaches maximum benefit

If you are new to doing intermittent fasting, you very well can have keto flu symptoms and/or be experiencing benefits outlined above in timeframes that happen sooner! Your body wants to feel better so once it is given support, it will GO TO WORK!

KETO FLU

When we intermittent fast, our body goes into something called ketosis!

We really are detoxing and cleansing, and this act literally is the body's version of the reset button on the back of your internet modem (are they still called modems?). That being said, in an article by Harvard Medical, it breaks down the phenomenon called The Keto Flu!

From the article: "The so-called keto flu is a group of symptoms that may appear two to seven days after starting a ketogenic diet. Headache, foggy brain, fatigue, irritability, nausea, difficulty sleeping, and constipation are just some of the symptoms of this condition, which is not recognized by medicine."

In addition to other symptoms like bad breath, stinky bowels and even skin rashes and acne, they don't know what causes keto flu but according to researchers like Suzanne Shaw and Paul Pitchford, these are a result of ...parasites, killing the parasites and then the elimination of said parasites; moreover, the parasites don't want to die! So we are at war with literal dark forces inside of us, and things can get a bit crazy in the body; however, fear not! The doctor-penned article goes on to state: "Do not give up if you are committed to a plan. You may feel exhausted for a few days, but at the end of a week, your energy level will most likely return to normal and you may feel even better." Those are words from a Harvard Medical Doctor!

So, if you feel the tea becoming overwhelming, stop drinking it for a couple days, while remaining true to every other part of the protocol...BUT, as you now know, be prepared to still have some Keto Flu symptoms arise, as the toxins and parasites leave your body.

EAT HIGH FREQUENCY FIBER-RICH SEASONAL PRODUCE & AVOID CERTAIN FOODS

When it comes to cleansing the body, the role of fiber-rich fruits and vegetables is primarily to support the body's natural detoxification processes. Fiber helps to move waste products through the digestive system more efficiently and can bind to toxins and promote their excretion from the body. Also, a diet rich in fruits and vegetables can provide a wide range of vitamins, minerals, and antioxidants that support the body's detoxification pathways and overall health.

Fiber-rich foods are beneficial for our health for several reasons:

Digestive health: Fiber helps to regulate bowel movements and prevents constipation by adding bulk to stool, which can promote regularity and prevent digestive issues.

Heart health: Diets high in fiber have been associated with a reduced risk of heart disease. Soluble fiber, in particular, can help lower LDL (low-density lipoprotein) cholesterol levels, also known as "bad" cholesterol, by binding to cholesterol and promoting its excretion.

Blood sugar management: Fiber can help regulate blood sugar levels by slowing down the absorption of sugar into the bloodstream. This can be particularly beneficial for individuals with diabetes or those at risk of developing diabetes.

Weight management: High-fiber foods are typically low in calories and can help promote satiety, or a feeling of fullness, which can help with weight management by reducing overall calorie intake.

Gut microbiota health: Fiber acts as a prebiotic, providing nourishment for beneficial bacteria in our gut, which can promote a healthy gut microbiota and overall gut health.

You will find a comprehensive list of fiber rich fruits and vegetables in *The Cellular Level* section of this book.

Avoid certain foods and beverages:

Meats, Fish (cooked and raw), Dairy, Eggs & Animal Products (This includes Chicken/Beef/Bone Broth), Processed foods, Canned Foods (Be careful with your consumption of canned fruits, vegetables, broth and soups! The high sodium will feed inflammation, increase blood pressure and costs you more energy to digest than it is giving you. Also - always rinse off your canned beans; however, only eat canned beans IF they are reduced sodium and cooked only in water, with no additional ingredients and preservatives! Opt instead to cook raw beans, lentils and legumes.), Seed Oils (Canola, Soybean, Corn, Sunflower, Safflower, Cottonseed, Grapeseed, Rice Bran), Fast food, Raw fish, Sugars (excluding fruits!), Refined carbohydrates (Pasta, Bread, Wheat, Gluten, White Flour); Alcohol should be avoided while on a detox regimen unless using a desired alcohol-based herbal tincture.

These foods and drinks can contribute to inflammation, congestion, disease and illness. Choosing to abstain from them does not have to be viewed as punishment; rather, see the temporary removal as an act of self-care, allowing the body to take a break and restore its natural balance.

FAQs

What order should I eat my food?

1. Vegetables

2. Fats and meats
3. Fruits and starches

Vegetables like peas, broccoli, etc contain both soluble and insoluble fiber, and when we eat vegetables first, the foods create this gooey-like mesh that covers our intestinal tracts. This is really beneficial because this natural layer is what will help the body correctly digest food. This gooey mesh helps the body from not quickly absorbing sugars and fats, while also creating a bit of a barrier where only enough of the good stuff breaks through, truly helping nutritional absorption.

When we eat, in a single meal, we should eat our veggies first, then fats and oils, then sugars and starches; moreover, this can truly be best applied to how we should go about eating throughout our day, especially those wanting to reverse their high blood pressure, high blood sugar and/or type 2 diabetes diagnosis.

So eating a breakfast of just vegetables turns the body into a TRANSFORMER! Now you're powering up the whole system for the day. Eat veggies in the morning, for lunch add in your fats and meats; moreover, it has also been stated that we shouldn't eat heavy proteins past 2p. For this, if we made lunch the time for consuming fats, oils and protein, keeping fruits and nuts for the afternoon as snacks and energy boosters, we are truly honoring our metabolism in the best ways possible!

Do I have to drink all of my Parasite Cleanse Tea and/or Cellular Detox Tea at once? Do I have to drink the 48oz of water recommended between 7a-11a and/or 11a-5p at one time?

No. You can prepare your teas first thing in the morning, and you have until 5p to drink the full daily amount (up to 32oz).

You have the full 3-hour (7a - 11a) and 6-Hour (11a - 5p) windows to drink the suggested amounts of water.

Is it okay to juice and/or make smoothies from fruits and vegetables?

Juicing fruits and vegetables and making smoothies can be considered forms of processing food, albeit in different ways, and they have implications for digestion and blood sugar regulation.

Juicing:

-Juicing involves extracting the liquid content from fruits and vegetables while leaving behind the pulp and fiber. This process removes much of the insoluble fiber, which is important for promoting satiety, regulating bowel movements, and slowing down the absorption of sugars into the bloodstream.

-Without the fiber, the natural sugars in fruits and vegetables are absorbed more rapidly into the bloodstream, leading to faster spikes in blood sugar levels. This rapid increase in blood sugar can subsequently result in energy crashes as blood sugar levels drop quickly after the initial spike.

-Furthermore, the absence of fiber in juice can also affect digestion. Fiber plays a crucial role in promoting healthy digestion by adding bulk to stool and supporting the growth of beneficial gut bacteria. Without sufficient fiber, digestive processes may be compromised, potentially leading to issues such as constipation.

Smoothies:

-Smoothies typically involve blending whole fruits and/or vegetables, including their fiber-rich skins or pulp, along with other ingredients such as liquids, nuts, seeds or protein powders. While smoothies retain more fiber than juices, the blending process still breaks down the fiber into smaller particles.

-While smoothies do provide more fiber compared to juices, the blending process can still lead to faster digestion and absorption of nutrients compared to consuming whole fruits and vegetables. This can result in quicker spikes in blood sugar levels, albeit to a lesser extent than with juices.

-Additionally, the act of blending can make the overall volume of food consumed in a smoothie more compact. This can potentially lad to consuming larger quantities of fruits and vegetables in a shorter period, which may overwhelm the digestive system and lead to discomfort for some individuals.

Is it really bad for me to add a smoked turkey leg to my pot of beans or greens?

This program specifically calls for a plant-based protocol...so yes...it is really that horrible to add a smoked turkey leg, and the reason is not torture your tastebuds!

Meat carries parasites, in addition to a host of other things. Adding a turkey leg is literally defeating the purpose of detoxing parasites from your body; moreover, the craving alone should make you question the need to 'dress up' raw and whole foods. These cravings, as you learn in the Circadian360 book, are potentially associated with parasites. Remember - every time you eat a food from the list of foods to avoid that are outlined in the Circadian360 Cellular Detox Protocol, you are feeding a parasite and thwarting your own progress. Your health, wellness and longevity are gifts that you must treasure as best you can, with the complete fullness of agency that you have over yourself.

I am so used to the unhealthy American breakfast with processed meats. Where should I get my protein from?

For sources of protein, you'll want to lean into lentils, chickpeas, quinoa, the many varieties of beans (cook your beans from scratch and avoid canned beans and canned foods in general). This is also a reason to add peas to many meals. There's 8g of protein in a single serving of peas! That's more protein than an egg! Most vegan protein powders leading ingredient are peas! So adding a couple servings to your morning salad and lunch salad replaces the 2 traditional eggs one would eat for breakfast or the 15-20g of lunch protein from fish or chicken.

Also consume the Circadian360 Vegan Chocolate Mushroom Protein Powder with 16g protein per serving, in addition to sustainably wild harvested mushrooms foraged directly from Mother Nature in the USA. A robust, all natural offering packing a wealth of nutritional benefits from nature's superfoods.

Is it okay for me to eat fruit in the morning for breakfast or as a snack?

Saving fruit consumption for the afternoons allows for the body to process and appreciate the usage and benefits of sugar so much more. Different regions and cultures are able to handle larger loads of fruits differently is because both the environment and their physical exertion allows for the metabolizing of the sugars in these foods to be directly converted to energy used for production. When we allow our bodies to not consume fruits until the afternoons, or at least later morning hours, we are also allowing for a slower absorption of the sugars, allowing for the potential boost in energy to carry us until the early evening.

Since we are avoid seed oils and the harmful traditional salad dressings, what can I use for salad dressing?

Fresh squeezed lemon and limes work well as a natural salad dressing, if needed. They also are astringent fruits that helps to support the digestive systems natural detoxification processes.

Why eat raw foods over cooked foods? Why avoid heating oils?

This protocol emphasizes the consumption of whole raw foods over cooked foods and advises against heating oils for health benefits and detoxification purposes due to several reasons. Firstly, raw foods retain their natural enzymes, vitamins, and minerals, which can be compromised or destroyed through cooking processes. These nutrients are essential for supporting various bodily functions and promoting overall health.

Additionally, heating oils can lead to the formation of harmful compounds such as trans fats, oxidized fats, and carcinogens, which may have adverse effects on cardiovascular health and contribute to inflammation in the body. By opting for raw foods and avoiding heated oils, your protocol aims to minimize exposure to these potentially harmful substances while maximizing the intake of nutrient-dense foods that support the body's natural detoxification processes. Raw foods are also often higher in fiber, which can aid digestion and promote the elimination of toxins from the body. Overall, prioritizing whole raw foods and minimizing the use of heated oils aligns with principles of natural, holistic nutrition and may contribute to improved health and vitality.

Your Light, Your Life: Closing Words

From the big picture to the cellular level, we've covered a treasure trove of wellness gems in this book, however, remember to take on the information in **Circadian360** with grace and balance, as you ascend towards a healthier and more authentic version of yourself.

In wisdom, we know that the only consistent fact about life is that it's always changing, and as light beings, this beautiful song is sung to us as a daily reminder when we honor the truth that the sun itself doesn't rise and set at the exact same time every day.

In this, we have an opportunity to accept that no matter what happens around us, when we rise each day to honor ourselves as light beings, we are choosing to exercise the best control, care and agency over our entire being, to the utmost of our abilities in that present moment. When we are living our lives and functioning at our highest respective individual states of optimal health, we are much more synchronized and aligned with the frequencies and vibrations of the world and universe around us, and in these intentional acts, we are *gifting* ourselves with the blessing of being much more prepared to both respond to and survive the factors outside of our control.

So each day, be gracious and treat yourself to wellness, finding joy in the inconsistencies that ultimately allow us opportunities to achieve growth and find balance.

Honor yourself through your "Non-Negotiable Lifestyle Routine", while compassionately remembering that *life happens.* In this, never become too strict and unwavering in your lifestyle that you're not able to be flexible with the up and down currents moving around you. For example, it certainly is unfortunate when your car breaks down and/or when you're in an vehicular accident; however, when you have insurance and/or financial protections to cover the damage, you're already approaching the circumstances equipped with tools to help both address and move on from the unfortunate situation far faster than if you weren't prepared.

So many factors in our day to day lives are outside of our control, and yet, the conscious circadian being authors their own epigenetic destiny, thriving with vitality and rejuvenation that can be traced back to their flourishing mitochondrial health and optimal levels of NAD+/longevity molecules. Through intentional acts, this conscious being understands that their existence illuminates far brighter when consuming a diet rich in high frequency foods, while keeping their behaviors, environments, clothings and choices aligned with the highest frequencies possible. Even reflected in their ascension of thoughts, these enlightened beings use neural synchronization to their advantage, as they seek and bond with others through brain waves in both intimate and social settings, becoming master architects and networkers building the worlds in which they choose to erect mentally and physically.

Through both my one on one and group coaching experiences, working intimately with individuals as they complete the **Circadian360 Cellular Detox Protocol**, upon completion of the program, for many, I find that it's akin to them stepping outside the confines of the Tibetan Wheel of Life for the first time.

The Tibetan Wheel of Life, deeply rooted in Buddhist philosophy, symbolizes the cycle of birth, death, and rebirth, perpetuated by our actions and desires. To step outside this wheel is to break free from the cyclical patterns of existence, to detoxify not just our bodies but also our minds and spirits.

Throughout history, the Wheel of Life has served as a reminder of the impermanence of life and the importance of making conscious choices to break free from harmful patterns. Through **Circadian360**, you're able to apply this energy towards understanding that each day becomes an opportunity for rebirth, a chance to navigate the amusements and dangers of life with increased awareness and wisdom. For some individuals, re-acclimating yourself with life outside of this program may bring about anxiety, as you're faced with situations of eating foods and/or engaging with and within spaces that you know are toxic and unhealthy for you.

What are you to do?

Don't take a step back!

Allow yourself to process the new data and information as what it is, recognizing just how far you've come. Ask yourself, is this conversation, experience, food and/or lifestyle choice contributing towards the vision of the person I am working to become? Whether if it is or isn't, be sure to then ask yourself WHY. The goal of this journey is to give you a fresh perspective on how you once were living, so that you can make the best choices moving forward that will be supportive of the life you deserve to lead.

The **Circadian360 Cellular Detox Protocol** is not to reset you to the point of being afraid of the amusements and amusement parks of life; rather, to emerge from the experience as a more aware and mindful human being who is consciously and intentionally living life as your best authentic expression of self, while maintaining as much agency and accountability over your own health as possible. I don't believe in living a human experience where we attempt to not be human (i.e, become so zen'd out that you are 'out of touch' with reality or so locked in on a eating protocol that you deny yourself a generous, home-cooked meal where the leading ingredient is love); however, I want us all to be able to return to life after following this detox protocol, with an awareness and more tools, allowing you to have agency over your own health and well-being!

Don't get so afraid of dairy that you deny yourself cake, but don't get so lost in the cake that you deny yourself optimum health and wellness, being fully aware of the work that you need to do, in order to healthily digest the food and properly eliminate the toxins from your body. When you find this divine balance...you really can have your own cake AND eat it too...and still look and feel so good tomorrow!

What if I need to take small steps? Just the thought of diving right in and following the entire Circadian360 Cellular Detox Protocol is overwhelming for me. What should I do and where should I start?

Research shows that information sticks when we write it down! So start by writing down:

1. Your vision of who you are going to become/the person that you know you are capable of being. Be as descriptive as possible - *How does your future self look? How does your future self feel?*

2. Write down your "WHYs" for becoming that person. Be as detailed as possible- *Why are you making these changes? Why can't you give up?*

You're doing this writing exercise because when you have a clear vision of where you are headed and it is supported with a clear knowing of why you are doing the work to fulfill that vision, you are prepared and equipped to face the unforeseen obstacles that may come. This initial task will become the spiritual fuel that you'll call upon, when deciding between the healthy and unhealthy choices that you're bound to face down the line.

Even if you don't change your diet, start upgrading your light! Follow the cosmic clock and create your own non-negotiable morning and evening routine, based on the circadian rhythm body clock. Allocate dedicated alone time for just you and the universe, in order to meditate, pray, give thanks, write goals, drink tea and watch the sunrise and sunset. This birthright, ancient ritual of being a human being connects us with the rhythms of our universe, reduces blood pressure, eases both stress and anxiety, builds the frontal lobe of the brain and gives us dedicated time to connect with the higher vibrations and sources of energies that are around us. Through these actions, we are able to positively strengthen the relationship that we each share in our interconnectedness with life itself.

Finally - invest in an old school alarm clock, strive to turn off your blue light emitting devices before 9 PM and stop sleeping with your smartphones in the same room! We must stop becoming such slaves to the false light that keeps both the brain and body constantly powered in a state of "On".

Again - **Circadian360** has equipped you with the tools and knowledge to approach each day as a new beginning, to make wiser decisions that align with your authentic self and aspirations. While the goal of the **Circadian360 Cellular Detox Protocol** isn't to instill fear of life's amusements, it is to foster mindfulness and intentionality in your journey towards optimal health and well-being.

By understanding the intricate workings of your circadian rhythm and embracing holistic strategies to harmonize with natural rhythms, you've unlocked the potential for profound healing and rejuvenation. From balancing light exposure to activating the Third Eye and flushing out toxins naturally, you've embarked on a path towards holistic wellness and vitality.

So go forth and live life as your most authentic, conscious circadian self, becoming the architect of your own well-being. Embrace your daily rituals as a canvas upon which you paint the hues of your aspirations, and remember to allocate time at the end of your day, week, month, season, and year for self-reflection and assessment. These moments of retrospective contemplation offer insights that pave the way for growth and evolution throughout your forthcoming days and seasons.

The time has now come for you to upgrade your quality of light, in order to improve the quality of your life! Disconnect from artificial light sources and devices emitting harmful EMFs. Step outside barefoot, feel the Earth's heartbeat, and let **Circadian360** be your guide as you 'turn off, unplug, and dance with the sun.'

Thank you for reading **Circadian360**. I invite you to join me at **Circadian360.com**, where additional tools and resources are available, to help you discover your solar blueprint, harness the power of sunlight and learn how to detoxify and rejuvenate your body, mind, and spirit on a cellular level.   - R.A. Massey

www.ingramcontent.com/pod-product-compliance
Lightning Source LLC
Chambersburg PA
CBHW080132270326
41926CB00021B/4445